Choosing Your Practice

Alan K. Kronhaus, M.D.

Choosing Your Practice

Springer-Verlag
New York Berlin Heidelberg
London Paris Tokyo Hong Kong

Alan K. Kronhaus, M.D.
Founder and CEO
KRON Medical
Clinical Faculty
Department of Medicine
University of North Carolina
Chapel Hill, North Carolina 27514, USA

Library of Congress Cataloging-in-Publication Data
Kronhaus, Alan K.
  Choosing your practice / Alan K. Kronhaus.
    p. cm.
  ISBN 0-387-97164-5
  1. Medicine—Practice. I. Title.
R728.K76 1990
610.69'52—dc20   89-39978

Cover concept by C. Maurer.
Typeset by Bytheway Typesetting Services, Norwich, New York.
Printed and bound by R. R. Donnelley & Sons Company, Harrisonburg, Virginia.
Printed in the United States of America.

9 8 7 6 5 4 3 2 1

ISBN 0-387-97164-5 Springer-Verlag New York Berlin Heidelberg
ISBN 3-540-97164-5 Springer-Verlag Berlin Heidelberg New York

This work is dedicated to:

*My parents, who made me believe I could do
whatever I set my mind to;
My wife, who is a constant source of
inspiration and strength;
and my colleagues, for whom I wrote the book.*

Preface

The realities of practicing medicine today make the need for this book compelling. The organizational landscape of medicine is changing with increasing speed as a result of the growing diversity of practice styles and professional opportunities. At the same time, many in the profession hesitate to acknowledge the importance of preparing physicians to function effectively in the real world.

There are few decisions we make as physicians that are more fundamental to our success and happiness than our choice of where, how, and with whom to practice. Ironically, there are few decisions we treat as cavalierly, at least as judged by the lack of time and effort we devote to choosing a practice wisely. Our failure to attend to a matter of such importance stems from the longstanding, deep-seated attitude within the profession that regards subjects such as career counseling and practice management as indecently vocational, unworthy of time on our educational agenda.

As dissatisfaction rises among physicians, the more responsible members of our profession are recognizing the need to help colleagues make their way in a world that appears increasingly hostile and hard to understand. For physicians, change within the healthcare industry, as in so many other areas of life, creates opportunities as well as anxieties. To capitalize on those opportunities, we must prepare for the challenges ahead.

This book might well have been titled "Everything You Always Wanted to Know About Choosing a Practice but Had No One to Ask About." My fondest hope is not only that it will fill an immediate need for information not previously available, but also that it will focus attention on the value of career counseling for physicians, an area that has long languished in the blind spot of professional education.

ALAN K. KRONHAUS, M.D.
Chapel Hill, North Carolina

Contents

Dilemmas of the Job Search

In setting the course of our careers, we as physicians make these major decisions: We choose medicine as an occupation, we select a specialty, and we decide where and how we want to practice. Most of us treat the first two decisions with due care and respect, but few of us seem to appreciate the importance of the third decision, at least as judged by the minimal time and attention we devote to choosing a practice wisely. The sobering fact that 50% of physicians change jobs during the first two years after training highlights how ill-prepared we are to choose a practice.

Why do so many of us fail to prepare properly for a decision of such importance? Until specialty training is complete, we generally find that others are making the major decisions concerning our lives: the courses and rotations we take, the clinics we cover, our call schedule and patient load—in essence, what we do and when we do it. Apart from choosing a medical school and postgraduate training program, we have little or no say in the formulation of our professional lives. Moreover, because professional commitments tend to dominate life during these years, we also have little control in the

---

Please note that this book is written with both women and men in mind. Forgive the author for simplifying matters by referring to physicians and all other personnel throughout the book as "he."

personal sphere. Not unfairly, one could characterize a physician's circumstances during this period as "sustained adolescence."

As a result, physicians experience a strange dichotomy in the structured, sheltered training environment. We exercise enormous responsibility for the welfare of others but have little control over much of what happens in our own lives. It is no wonder, then, that when it comes time to choose where and how to practice, we shy away from making such a major life decision. If indeed we make mistakes at this point and do not learn from those mistakes, our subsequent career moves or life decisions may produce equally poor results.

Who is to blame for these unfortunate circumstances? One school of thought places the responsibility at the doorstep of those in the medical profession who dictate what is learned in medical school and postgraduate training. These individuals, who might very well have provided career guidance and counseling to the young physicians for whom they are making many other life decisions, have abdicated their responsibilities in this vital area. This book is part of a growing effort on the part of the more responsible members of the profession to redress a glaring oversight: failure to prepare physicians to function effectively in the real world.

To make matters worse, there is considerable pressure to choose a practice correctly the first time. The stakes are particularly high for two reasons. First, most of us are considerably older than the rest of the population when we seek our first "real" job. We have invested more in our education and have often accumulated enormous debts. Moreover, we have generally married and so have extensive social and family commitments. Second, although changing jobs, like getting divorced, has become more socially acceptable, it still carries a stigma. Other physicians tend to be wary of a prospective partner who has moved several times. There is thus but a small margin of error in regard to making a false start or similar mistake. Multiple practice changes engender great hardship for the physician and grave misgivings among his peers.

State of Medicine Today

Today the medical profession offers its practitioners an almost limitless diversity of professional opportunities, many of which were not available until the decade of the 1980s. This diversity of choice, as in many other areas of life, is associated with both good news and bad news. The good news is that the probability of finding a practice well suited to the needs and personality of the job-seeker is greater than ever before, which unfortunately gives rise to the bad news: the greater likelihood of a major mismatch.

Choosing an appropriate practice in a situation that may at first seem enveloped in chaos and confusion calls for a reasonable, logical approach. Such an approach, offered in this book, boils down to fitting a round peg in a round hole. It starts with a guide to self-assessment that will help you understand yourself and the practice environment in which you will thrive. It then goes on to provide vital information for the second half of the equation: What types of practice are available? What are their advantages and disadvantages? The book also highlights key questions that should be asked of one's self and of future associates or employers. Finally, it suggests ways to match the hopes and desires of the job seeker with the most suitable opportunity available.

Given the complexity of human nature and the countless medical practices within reach, one cannot write a "how-to" book with facile answers. This volume, however, does provide a framework that will help you explore opportunities and position yourself optimally in your chosen profession.

The trend toward increasing diversity of practice styles offers marvelous opportunities. It is just a matter of being willing to prepare for and persist in finding the ideal practice. It is said that *discovery comes to the prepared mind*. It was with this thought that the book was conceived and written.

Neophyte Physicians and Their Mistakes

One night you decide that it is time to get married. You go to the local disco and dance once or twice with the best looking members of the opposite sex. By the end of the evening, based on your experience, you choose the lucky man or woman with whom you plan to spend the years to come.

Ridiculous as this scenario seems, it is frighteningly close to the way many of us choose our practice and our professional associates. Someone once said that a partnership is like a marriage without sex. Imagine how difficult it would be to make a success of that kind of relationship. The probability of success is even more limited when the time and effort are not sufficient at the beginning to find out what you are getting into. The fact is that most of us have little information and even less experience to guide us when choosing a practice. We know little about opportunities available and the advantages and disadvantages of each. It is no wonder that the turnover in medical practice is high.

Many of us do not know what we are looking for in the first place. Among the 17,000 doctors completing their training each year, probably one-half to two-thirds spin the wheel of fortune when it comes to choosing their practice and accept an appointment wherever it stops.

The result is that countless physicians arrive each morning at a practice for which they are ill-suited and in which they cannot be happy. Countless others have been through false starts and relocations. The dissatisfaction that accrues from such situations is a bitter pill considering the educational and temporal investment made in getting to that point. Is it any wonder, then, that on almost any scale of discontent or malaise—stress, depression, burnout, divorce, substance abuse, suicide—physicians are at or near the top of the national statistics?

What is most surprising is that we physicians—bright, well-educated people—having gone through intensive training in patient management and rational thinking, virtually abdicate reason when it comes to one of the major steps in our lives, the critically important task of choosing a practice. Is this problem a variation on the theme that "doctors make the worst patients"?

This discussion is not suggesting that an unsuitable practice is the sole cause of unhappiness among physicians. Some of us entered medical school with little understanding of what being a doctor is all about. We envisioned an exciting career studded with difficult cases and high drama but have wound up stitching minor cuts, treating sniffles, and stroking the worried well.

Some of us chose the wrong specialty. Some oncologists wind up being more depressed than they expected; some pediatricians grow bitter over the disparity in income among the specialties; and some obstetricians cannot handle being sued for every bad outcome (e.g., the mother who decides that her baby's' failure to score 1200 on the

SAT is due to heretofore unrecognized brain trauma sustained at birth). Others of us dislike the politics and paperwork inherent in any form of practice, and yet others despair over the waning of professional sovereignty.

There are many reasons some of us wind up unhappy as physicians. The fundamental premise of this book is that a poorly chosen, ill-fitting practice underlies more of the unhappiness and discontent in the profession than we have acknowledged. It is unlikely that the physician who is unhappy at work will feel compensated by the money earned or the privileges, accomplishments, and prestige gained as a professional. Choosing a practice wisely, then, is the key to professional satisfaction and a decent return on the educational investment made.

This book is about exactly that—how to choose a practice thoughtfully, rationally, and intelligently. It provides guidance and information to fill the gap left by our medical schools and postgraduate training programs when they neglected the issues of career counseling and practice management, considering them "indecently vocational" and therefore unworthy of time on the curriculum.

Considering the experiences of physicians who have "been through it" is a valuable way to examine these issues. Some of the physicians whose stories are told below were just starting out, and others had been through traumatic experiences before. Each was well credentialed and well intentioned. Their stories are told so you can learn from their mistakes, all of which could have been avoided by intelligent legwork and thoughtful questioning before they decided where to settle and establish a practice.

"Case" Studies

REBOUNDING

Michelle had been through a very tough, very good training program. She had been constantly reminded that "giants strode these halls." She had experienced three years of long hours, endless obligations, critical cases, and complex problems with little time off—all with the idea of maximizing her clinical experience.

Toward the end of the program, she was forced to turn her attention to finding a practice. Everyone (parents, friends, colleagues, faculty) expected her to find something suitably "blue chip" to validate her elite education. Drained and exhausted by the pressures of the rigorous program, she overreacted in the opposite direction.

She turned down several tenure track academic positions as well as offers to work with large, prestigious groups. "Too demanding," she thought. She coveted regular hours, time to herself, time for shopping, time to be a woman, and maybe time to marry and start a family. When she stopped to examine her attitudes, she was surprised at how wide-ranging her thoughts were. She realized that she needed time to get her bearings in life.

She accepted an offer to work in a walk-in clinic in a neighborhood shopping center. This situation would cause no undue pressures, she reasoned. The pay was decent, and, more importantly, the schedule was easy. Regular, predictable hours and an accommodating staff to help at every turn—the exact opposite of her training experience. She could even schedule her time to include long weekends.

As far as her schedule and workload went, the practice was truly all that it had promised. In fewer than three months, however, she was weary of suturing minor lacerations and treating sore throats. After the interesting cases she had dealt with during her training, this walk-in work was boring.

To make matters worse, she got little satisfaction from doctor-patient relationships, which rarely went beyond a single encounter. The interesting cases were referred to better equipped private physicians who rarely referred the patients back; the acute cases were sent to the hospitals, from which there was no feedback unless she took the initiative to follow up.

Michelle had not realized how quickly she could become disenchanted with clinical work and her role as a physician. She had not recognized that what she needed was a middle-of-the-road practice, something with a patient load and case mix half-way between crazy-intense and maddeningly dull.

Her next move was to a closed-panel health maintenance organization (HMO), which provided her with a group of patients close to the number and type she wanted. Unfortunately, she soon found the HMO too large, bureaucratic, and cold. At least at the walk-in clinic she was treated like someone important. At the HMO she was a cog in the wheel, more a functionary than an influence in the practice. In fact, she called herself the "doctor machine" because that is the way she was treated—like one of the machines the clinic tried to keep going with the minimum necessary maintenance. She had little or no input on anything; her opinions were never solicited and, when given, were rarely considered. Mothballing intelligence is no easy proposition for such a bright person.

Summation. Michelle now knows that she does not want an ultra-high-intensity practice that recreates her training experience, nor does she desire a mundane practice that fails to draw on any part of her previous experience. This recognition came at a cost of three years, two major moves, and two emotional jolts—because she had not defined what she wanted in the first place.

If you fail to develop a clear idea of what you are looking for, you are liable to overreact to current circumstances. We all want to make decisions that do not repeat past problems and deficiencies. Decisions made on that basis, however, can easily swing you from one set of problems to another, passing over that all-important "middle ground" where the "right spot" often lies.

Michelle should have begun a thoughtful consideration of the issues early in her residency, well before the pressure to choose a practice began to crescendo. Had she planned her career in that way, the facts on which she would base her decisions would be in reasonable focus, in perspective, when it came time for her to act.

EXTERNAL POLITICS

David was recruited out of his residency by the senior partner of a three-doctor anesthesiology group. He was to replace an associate who had recently departed because of a divorce. Everything about the setup seemed right: It was a fee-for-service group with a solid record of high income and good relationships with local surgeons. The practice seemed well managed. He would be made a full partner after a brief six-month trial, with no buy-in.

Unfortunately, there was more going on than met the eye, even in this apparently tranquil, bucolic setting. Three weeks after he started, David found that his new associates were embroiled in an emotion-packed conflict with the administrator of the town's 150-bed hospital. The administrator was new in town, having been hired when a hospital management chain took over operation of the facility a year before David appeared on the scene.

The administrator believed that anesthesiologists should be salaried hospital employees, and he was pressuring David's group to forsake its fee-for-service arrangement for the salaried positions he had already forced the radiologists and pathologists to accept. The group resisted, whereupon the administrator hired a new anesthesiologist, gave him an exclusive contract for anesthesia services at the hospital, and revoked the hospital privileges of the members of David's group.

The group went to court not three months after David's arrival. This situation was a shock for David, who was so unfamiliar with legal matters that he had not even asked an attorney to review his employment agreement.

Nine months, two injunctions, and $150,000 in legal fees later, the group prevailed, surviving in the meantime on its receivables. When their privileges were restored, David and his associates were able to resume practice on their own terms, but things were still not well. David was now competing with one more anesthesiologist than the small town could support, and the hospital administrator was more committed than ever to the group's demise.

Enraged over the legal defeat, the administrator put subtle but persistent pressure on the town's surgeons to utilize the salaried anesthesiologist-employee. They succumbed; and although there was enough overflow to support David's two partners, there was not enough to keep David's practice active. It was also obvious that, in time, the administrator would add another salaried anesthesiologist, then another, until David's beleaguered colleagues were starved out.

An honorable fellow, David left on his own rather than force his partners to split a two-person income three ways. Unknowingly, David had joined a practice that was already in the administrator's gun sights, and he took the first hit.

Summation. David took a look at the practice, liked what he saw, and believed he had done his homework. He signed on because he "felt good" about the practice and the community, seeing the situation as one in which he could thrive. He was right, as far as he went.

A practice—like any organization or organism, for that matter—exists in and interacts with its environment. Its success, indeed its viability, depends on its ability to cope with its changing external environment as well as its internal affairs.

David simply did not look deeply or thoroughly enough into the external factors that were likely to affect his practice. He looked around, liked what he saw on the surface, and stopped short of asking even the few basic questions that would have revealed the problem he subsequently encountered.

LIFE STYLE MISTAKE

Doug and Jeff were best friends through medical school and post-graduate training. Both internists, they presumed they would practice together long before either of them broached the subject. Without giving it much thought, each assumed that their compatibility as friends would translate into compatibility as partners.

It was not to be the case. Doug and Jeff were marching to different drummers. Jeff was the dedicated type who would have been happy in Mongolia so long as he could practice good medicine and help people. His wife, who had known him since junior high school, had grown up with his dreams, understood his career, and supported him fully.

Doug had never married. He, too, was dedicated, but, unlike Jeff, he thought there was more to life than medicine. He enjoyed working, but he wanted his free time as well, planning to fill it with exciting people and interesting recreation. A demanding practice would be a sacrifice for him in terms of life style. However, he set his personal preferences aside in order to practice with the more zealous, driven Jeff. Doug was also the more dollar-conscious of the two, so he was eager to build a lucrative practice and become financially successful.

Doug and Jeff set up a two-man practice in a quiet, upper class suburb. Business was slow at first, naturally, and the two spent enormous amounts of time developing a patient base: speeches at the Rotary club, trips to the emergency room to treat minor problems, assiduous follow-up on all new patients, medical advice articles for the local newspaper, even the occasional house call.

Through it all, Jeff had strong support at home. Knowing him so long and so well, his wife, a registered nurse, was inured to the routine and was prepared for the sacrifices. Doug would like to have been married, but until the right woman happened along, he would enjoy the single life—at least he would have if he could have found the time.

After nearly two years, the situation seemed perfect—professionally. The work was finally paying off, and the practice had become well established. Jeff and his wife had a baby, and their dreams seemed to be coming true. Doug, however, was struggling. As the practice grew, it took more of his time than ever, as more patients meant more hours, more calls, and less personal time. The money was great, but every other night and every other weekend were given over to work. He had no time to enjoy himself, and he was usually too tired anyway. There was no spouse to provide support, and he had no time to look for one. Even his apartment was depressing. He was still living with orange crates because he had had no time to furnish it properly.

"Why am I doing this?" he finally asked himself. He suddenly realized that he had not thought through what he was looking for at this stage of his life, had not acknowledged that he really did not want to work this hard. It also began to dawn on him that he had been influenced by the lure money and his friendship with Jeff, who was able to sustain himself on dedication and zeal.

Two friends had chosen a practice that appeared at first to accommodate both. Indeed it worked well for Jeff, who had his workload and was happy with the money. Doug, however, although financially secure, felt that the workload was wrecking his life.

Summation. When choosing a practice, Doug took the easy way out. He hitched his wagon to Jeff's, and he focused on one issue—money—instead of analyzing his overall goals, values, and preferences. Tackling the big picture is difficult, but avoiding the tough questions leaves you vulnerable. This juncture of life is no place to take the easy way out.

Doug and Jeff wound up in a practice that suited Jeff perfectly but Doug not at all, except for the money, which turned out not to be enough to compensate for a life that was otherwise miserable. With no wife to support him and no desire to settle down, his personal needs clashed with his professional commitments.

If you do not make a concerted effort to "know yourself," you are not likely to find a professional situation that resonates with who you are and what you want out of life. The process of getting to know yourself requires that you candidly consider and balance many factors, not focus on just one. (This subject is covered thoroughly in Chapter 3.)

POISONED COMMUNITY

The hospital administrator in a small New England town recruited Martin, a young obstetrician, by describing the unmet demand created recently when the town's two obstetricians left. "You can fill the void," he was told, "and your practice will hit the ground running."

Intrigued, Martin went for an on-site interview. He found the few townsfolk he spoke with pleasant, the quaint, rustic setting lovely, and the health care professionals clearly supportive of his joining them.

Martin had always envisioned himself in a relatively small community, a place where he could be an important person. He was not afraid of the workload that comes with a solo obstetrics practice. Thus he moved in and set up an office.

After several weeks of a slow start in the community, Martin became aware of the reasons his predecessors, one male and one female had left. It seems that the male predecessor had had an affair with a patient, creating a scandal that eventually had forced him to leave.

The female obstetrician was then saddled with the town's entire obstetrics practice, which quickly exhausted her. Moreover, she felt tainted by the scandal and by the town's negative image of physicians in her specialty, even though she was guilty of nothing. Within six months of her colleague's departure, she threw in the towel and moved 20 miles away to a larger town. It was a new location and a new start, and she was comforted by the notion that fewer people paid attention to her business.

Meanwhile, back in the scandalized community, Martin found himself dealing with the fear and animosity of the few patients who came to his office. Half of the women in town had reconciled themselves to driving the 20 miles to remain with the obstetrician with whom they were familiar, and the other half were afraid to consult a male obstetrician, fearing sexual advances. In short, young Martin starved, despite his eagerness to do well, work hard, be well liked, and contribute to the town and to society in general.

Summation. Like David in the vignette above, Martin did not evaluate the myriad "environmental" and contextual factors—economic, social, political, medical, historical, cultural—likely to affect his practice. As we are seeing, a few focused questions can glean crucial information about the realities of a practice situation.

Can you imagine trying to care for patients without taking a proper history? It is clear that we can obtain the information we need from a patient once we understand the proper questions to ask. One of the goals of this book is to help you appreciate the issues you need to look into and the questions you need to ask to properly evaluate a given opportunity.

"An ounce of prevention is worth a pound of cure." Never was this cliche more applicable. Certainly it takes time to look into things thoroughly; but with such care, you will be handsomely compensated by the effort and aggravation you are spared later.

INTERNAL POLITICS

Jean, an internist, joined a large multispecialty group in a suburban town, population 35,000. She had been assured that there was plenty of work, and indeed there was. She saw patients virtually from morning to night, some 65 hours a week. At the end of her first year she had earned $85,000, somewhat more than she had expected. Jean was fairly pleased with herself, thinking that it was a pretty nice start in life.

She could not shake a nagging discontent, however, that had begun about halfway through the first year when she realized that the group's radiologists made about $150,000 with a 8:00 a.m. to 3:00 p.m. schedule, a half-day off during the week, and no call duty.

Checking further, she had found that the group's anesthesiologists made $200,000, minimum, for even less time at work.

Jean asked the administrator for a look at the group's rules for dividing revenue. She was astonished to find the rules heavily favoring the consultative and procedure-oriented specialists who, after all, depended on their primary-care colleagues for referrals but shared none of their on-call responsibilities. They earned double the money and more! Jean came to view the physician roster in terms of first- and second-class citizens and was furious over recognizing herself in the lower tier.

To make matters worse, the group's doddering elder statesman practiced almost no medicine but was paid handsomely for the speeches he delivered and the public relations functions he attended. He made the same speeches to the same groups in the same good ol' boy network year after year. He earned more money for playing 18 holes of golf than Jean did for 10 hours of seeing patients. Jean also discovered that certain group members were paid extra for their role in the state medical society, and others drew additional compensation for articles they published. Where, she asked, is the equity?

Jean set about trying to solve a dilemma that had undone countless physicians before her: She suggested to the group's executive committee that physicians get paid extra for coming into the hospital when they are on call. Predictably, the radiologists and referral physicians in the group squawked, from the dermatologist to the plastic surgeon, arguing that call duty was part of being a physician, not something that warrants specific compensation. "Not a bad position to take," thought Jean, "if you seldom take call and rarely get disturbed when you do."

Jean was accused of trying to create a revenue source for herself and the other primary care physicians. The referral physicians complained that if such a change came about they would not have a crack at that type of income. Jean offered them as much of her call as they wanted. Not unexpectedly, they wanted no part of it. The referral and the procedure-oriented physicians in the group thus became incensed at what appeared to be a flagrant attempt to alter the group's income distribution policy. The showdown came when the radiologists and anesthesiologists, along with a handful of the referral physicians, threatened to walk out if the Board approved Jean's "new and improved" income distribution proposals.

The outcome was as inevitable as it was economic. The town was shorter on radiologists and anesthesiologists than it was on internists and family physicians, and the prospect of recruiting hospital-based specialists was even more bleak than it was for recruiting primary care physicians. Jean, a young professional full of principles, could not live with the inequity and the unfairness. She walked out of the meeting and out of the group.

Summation. Methods of dividing income vary and are often a major source of dissension in multispecialty groups, particularly those that include widely divergent specialties with large disparities in income potential. Jean was naive and ill-informed. She had wanted to join a multispecialty group for many valid reasons, but this issue and its importance should have been one of her considerations when she interviewed with her potential employers.

Because such disparities are part and parcel of multispecialty group practice, Jean must come to terms with the realities of the situation and decide the degree of income disparity she can tolerate. The referral physicians in the group she chose did not create the disparity; they simply benefited from it. If Jean cannot accept the inclination of other specialists to capitalize on market realities, she should opt for a practice where such differences are less pronounced, e.g., academic practice, single-specialty groups, the military, large HMOs.

CULTURE CLASH

Henry was a city boy. Born and raised in New York, he went to medical school there and then on to an anesthesiology residency in neighboring New Jersey. "Gettin' owtta New Yawk" had been Henry's goal for some time, and when he received a breathtaking financial offer from a small hospital in rural Georgia he was happy beyond words.

In the small town that recruited him, he became a one-man department, with the help of certified registered nurse anesthetists (CRNAs). He worked Monday through Friday, seldom on weekends, and was home early every afternoon. He and his wife spent much of their spare time designing and overseeing the construction of a palatial house, easily the finest, best appointed house the area had ever seen. It cost nearly $500,000, but his income could easily support it.

Once the house was finished, however, Henry and his wife found little else to amuse them. Atlanta was too far for a simple evening out, and there was no appropriate social life for them in the area, no one to whom they could relate. Henry and his neighbors gave each other culture shock, and so he and his wife soon felt isolated. They went so far as to have much of their food shipped in from Balducci's (specialty grocer) in New York, as the local fare did not satisfy their gastronomic (and perhaps psychological) needs.

The slow pace of life, especially at the hospital, began to tell on both of them. It came to the point where Henry, the New Yorker, could barely relate even to the rest of the medical staff, southerners all. What was worse, he had locked himself into the practice—into a one-man show, where that one man gets no time off unless he can arrange coverage, and Henry could not.

Turning increasingly inward, Henry and his wife made their home a virtual recreation center. They bought all the electronic equipment an audiophile could want, enough exercise equipment for world class athletes, and every amusing gadget from every catalogue they could lay their hands on. It did not help.

After three years, they had had enough. Henry went job hunting in New York, but his resume raised questions everywhere. He lacked colleagues who would attest to his current competence. Skeptical New Yorkers wondered how anyone in his right mind could go to rural Georgia, and they were suspicious about what had happened that he had not "made it" there. In contract negotiations, he had to give in on every point. He was forced to take hours of continuing medical education, for example, as his rural hospital had been too small for complex surgery and had handled no obstetrics or pediatric cases.

It became increasingly apparent that the demand for anesthesiologists was not the same in New York as it was in rural Georgia and that he was negotiating from a deficit position. Finally, he settled for 50% of what he had been making and felt fortunate to get it.

Henry listed his house for $850,000, but no one in the area could afford such a place. He finally sold it for $300,000, just to stop paying $4500 a month interest on his $450,000 mortgage. By the time he was done paying the first and last months' rent plus a security deposit for his New York apartment (which incidentally was smaller than his former game room) Henry had virtually nothing to show for his three years of hard work and high income in Georgia.

Summation. Choosing a practice is a matter of weighing numerous factors. Henry had focused on only two: getting out of New York and making a great deal of money. Prominent among the factors he failed to consider were the cultural, social, and recreational aspects of the community he was to call home. Moreover, he virtually ignored the effect the move would have on his wife.

He might have avoided the mistakes he made and the price he paid, financial and otherwise, if he had taken a broader view of himself and what he was getting into. Ideally, he could have tested his choice by doing locum tenens in that community or a similar one. Having not tested the waters, Henry should not have dived in head first.

If you are foolish enough to rush forward without knowing what lies ahead, at least leave yourself an easy way out. It is best not to paint yourself into a corner with a long-term contract or by making financial commitments to a fancy office or a large home.

PHILOSOPHICAL CLASH

Duncan trained in one of the country's oldest, best, and most respected institutions where he had been inculcated with the ethic that a doctor spares no time, effort, and certainly no expense for even the most minor benefit to the patient. After training, he went to his wife's home town of Minneapolis and joined the staff of a large HMO. After only three weeks on the job, he was called into the business manager's office to discuss his "style of practice," specifically the number of tests he had been ordering. In a nutshell, the manager suggested that he make fewer expenditures and practice with a much sharper eye on the bottom line. "Each account—er, patient—is supposed to generate a profit, not a loss, for the practice," he was told. Four weeks later the manager repeated the lecture, this time with considerably less friendliness and much more urgency.

In time, Duncan found himself "going along" in order to "get along." He began making unsavory tradeoffs—bypassing laboratory tests or short-changing patients on the counseling and reassurance he once considered so important. It was not long before he became disgusted with his own behavior, and he began to look elsewhere for employment.

"At Mudville Medical Center we never discourage doctors from ordering any test or performing any procedure that's in the best interest of the patient," the medical director told him. Mozart could not have written better music for Duncan's idealistic ears. He signed on.

In fact, Mudville Medical Center did not discourage Duncan from ordering whatever he wanted. Just the opposite—he soon realized that he was being encouraged, indeed pushed and pressured to order tests, irrespective of appropriateness and propriety. The practice, you see, had elaborate, expensive in-house laboratory and imaging facilities that the doctors were expected to "feed." Members of the group were thus ordering baseline tests for every possible condition, were "screening" for the most exotic disorders, and were repeating tests with unexplained frequency. It was no wonder that the revenue from ancillary services represented 65% of the group's income.

Duncan's colleagues were even performing risky procedures for which they were minimally trained, thereby avoiding referral outside the group. It became obvious to Duncan that the driving force in this practice was the partners' pocketbooks, not the patients' best interest. Sadly, Duncan was soon job hunting again.

Summation. Duncan had not made the intellectual adjustment from the protected environment of residency to the real world. In the real world, medicine is more than an exercise in patient care; it is a business. If you do not make money for the practice, your tenure will be limited.

Such a situation is not necessarily bad for the patient, but it can be. As a principled physician committed to the patient's best interests, you had better determine what financial pressures are likely to be placed on you in one or another type of practice. Working in several practices for short periods is the best way to understand these pressures and how you respond to them; talking to colleagues and asking pointed questions can also help. However you go about it, you should develop your own philosophy or style of practice, a key element of which is your inclination to err in the direction of over- or under-ordering tests, assuming that a perfect balance is difficult to achieve. The sensible choice of practice is one in which the financial incentives are in harmony with the way you prefer to practice.

NOT READY TO SETTLE DOWN

As Mark was approaching the last few months of medical residency, fellow residents, faculty, parents, and friends incessantly asked him, "What are you going to do next year?" What Mark really wanted was some time off, a career break. There were so many things he wanted to do. His secret desire was to be a wildlife photographer, although everyone else had high expectations for him in medicine. He also wanted to travel before settling down; it was part of his motivation for undertaking wildlife photography—to visit exotic places, hike to high plateaus, camp out in a tent, linger at will. He felt that if he just had the time to relax and wait for that "perfect picture" he would be a happy man.

One day, quite by accident, he met the head of a four-man pediatrics group that had room for a fifth. "It's not really what I want to do," Mark thought, "but if I take it I won't have to worry about what to do or where the money will come from." A few weeks, several calls, and one interview later he signed on.

"Oh, well" thought Mark, "I've kept my nose to the grindstone this long, what's another few years." He rationalized his decision by saying that he could establish himself now and catch up with his dreams later. He would have more money to pursue photography then anyway.

Soon Mark was in practice, again doing what people expected of him. He learned the ropes quickly and soon became a productive member of the group. Before long, he acquired a wife and baby, a house, the traditional responsibilities, and all the respect his community could offer. He was so locked in to this life that he could not imagine a free weekend outdoors, let alone a week's excursion into the wilderness. He kept his nonmedical interest alive by subscribing to every photography magazine published, but the only photographs he took were those of this child growing up.

Year after year things looked brighter and brighter—by everyone else's standards. Mark made more and more money, accumulated more and more belongings, sat on more and more committees. Inside, however, Mark was growing more and more discontented.

He tried talking about it to his colleagues. Completely absorbed in medicine, they did not take him seriously. Not one of his co-workers could imagine "fooling around" with something outside of medicine. His wife took him seriously, though, and became alarmed, although not for the right reasons: She was terrified of insects, hated to hike, and became claustrophobic in even the most spacious backpacker's tent.

Thoroughly confused and with no one to talk to, Mark became increasingly anxious. He began to have trouble falling asleep at night and then, once he finally got to sleep, woke up several times before morning. He remembered from his college days that marijuana made him sleepy, so he started smoking it again for the first time in twelve years. It seemed to help—for a while. Soon, no matter how stoned he got, he woke up two hours after falling asleep and nearly every hour thereafter. He turned to sleeping pills, the old-fashioned barbiturate type. They worked better and made him feel better. Soon Mark was hooked.

Summation. There is more to life than the practice of medicine. The personal dimensions of your life are as important, as much a part of you, as the professional part. If you ignore who you are and what you want outside of medicine, it ultimately catches up with you.

The socialization process in medicine is so powerful and the time requirements so rigorous that we are sorely tempted to focus solely on what is expected of us as physicians. With only a single focus, we are in a precarious position, balancing our lives on one pillar. No career, not even the most successful, progresses perfectly. When something goes wrong professionally, as it inevitably does, we need something to smooth out the wrinkles. Everyone is subject to disappointments, setbacks, frustrations. Some of us fall back on family, and some rely on a hobby. It does not matter what it is, so long as there is something and it is kept well integrated in your life and your plans for the future.

Once you abdicate the personal dimension of your life—if you do not pursue what is important to you apart from medicine—you leave a void that tends to be filled by any one of a number of unpleasant substitutes. In Mark's case it was barbiturates.

REVOLVING DOOR

Sheldon accepted a job offer that included a higher-than-expected starting salary and a shorter-than-expected waiting period to partnership and profit sharing. Other key elements of the package were generous as well: The limits of his malpractice insurance were higher than he thought were needed, and the group leased a car for him. His compensation over the first three years of employment exceeded that offered to any of his fellow residents, and he could hardly wait to sign the contract.

He had shown the contract to a friend for some casual feedback, and the friend expressed some discomfort that it did not clearly specify the terms and conditions governing the group's final decision on granting partnership status. "I can see what you're saying," Shelley said, "but you haven't met these people. They're real nice guys. I trust them."

Thus Sheldon never asked them how they decided on granting partnership or even about the basis for termination. He never looked into malpractice tail provisions or the group's history with other junior associates. How many had become partners over the last five years? Sheldon was afraid that even raising the issue would signal a lack of trust to his prospective associates. He decided "not to look a gift horse in the mouth" and accepted the offer with all its vagueness.

Much to Shelley's satisfaction, the group came through with everything it promised—until year three, when the group voted against granting him partnership. His world caved in. Not only did he not realize the expected gain from his share of the profits, he had to purchase tail coverage for his malpractice policy (it was a whooping 150% of his annual premium) and pick up the remaining payments on his car lease. Worse, there was a restrictive covenant in the contract precluding him from establishing a separate practice within miles of that community.

He was thus forced to move, with all its accompanying expenses. He was unable to sell his house immediately, and nearly went bankrupt before he finally reestablished a cash flow to cover these unforeseen, unplanned-for expenses.

Summation. Sheldon did not know what he was getting into. Any deal "too good to be true" probably is. To evaluate an offer adequately, you must ask the right questions of the right people; and with experience and knowledge, this exercise is not difficult.

Contractual details are important, particularly those related to the term and renewal of the contract, compensation, termination, ownership, profit sharing, malpractice insurance, indemnification, and noncompetition. Nitpicking is unnecessary, but ignoring what is important is foolhardy. Never be afraid to ask questions and discuss issues you consider important with the person or persons hiring you.

Defining the Problem

Your colleagues in the vignettes just outlined are not exceptions; they are the rule. Typically, young job hunting physicians believe the profession is waiting to welcome them, and older, experienced physicians are sure their colleagues are anxious to utilize the years of experience they offer. Each of us expects to be received warmly and treated professionally in the marketplace. No wonder many of us walk straight into disappointment and sometimes disaster.

Choosing a practice is a career decision as important as any you have made or will make. It is as important as choosing medicine as an occupation or deciding on a specialty. Unfortunately, most of us are decidedly ill-prepared to choose a practice wisely.

At the point we complete our training, we have little or no idea of what is beyond the academic "iron curtain." We are forced to make a major life decision with little insight into what pleases or displeases us, little knowledge of the professional opportunities available, and poor understanding of their advantages and disadvantages. We have had few real world role models and even fewer courses or words of advice to guide us. In other words, we have little or no basis for making one of the most important decisions of our lives.

To make matters worse, we have functioned throughout medical school and postgraduate training in highly structured situations—as already noted, in a state of "sustained adolescence." Aside from choosing a medical school and a residency program, we have had to think little about what we want to do or where we want to go with our lives. We have had only to stay afloat.

When we make the transition from training to private practice or from one practice to another, however, we must deal with a great many issues. We must suddenly establish a direction and structure to our lives, and we are poorly prepared to do that.

Bad News/Good News

Our training programs have not addressed real world issues such as choosing a practice or managing one. Ostrich-like, those responsible for the curriculum stick their heads in the sand when it comes time to help younger colleagues make key career decisions. The net effect is that we physicians complete the ritual of schooling and training only to find ourselves unprepared to function successfully in the real world.

Not uncommonly, we deal with this dilemma by postponing our departure from the nest. How many of us accept fellowships simply because they are there? At some point, though, we can no longer rationalize another year of training, another degree or credential. Not knowing how to go about choosing a practice, we often accept the first position offered. This lack of discrimination often results in a mistake.

If that is the bad news, the good news is that many such mistakes are avoidable. We do not have to start over or take graduate level courses in life planning or career management. This book can help by providing guidelines with which you can gather the essential information. More importantly, it provides a framework within which you can gain insight from your own experiences. It can put you in a position to direct your own career despite the lack of preparation you have suffered up to this point.

■ 2

The Costs of Career Mistakes

The cliche that mistakes are expensive applies to the process of choosing a practice. However, because many physicians do not think in economic terms, we tend to underestimate or ignore the costs of our career mistakes. This attitude is unfortunate because the stakes are high.

The cost of choosing the wrong practice takes three forms. First, there are the *hard costs*—the money spent on items such as moving, buying a house or furnishing an apartment, outfitting an office, and becoming established in a community. Added to these costs are professional fees for lawyers, accountants, and other business consultants.

Second, there are the *opportunity costs*—the difference between what is and what might have been. When you buy a car, for example, the hard costs are enumerated on the sticker; the opportunity cost is the return you might have realized on an alternative investment—the 7% you might have made on municipal bonds, for example. In terms of career mistakes, "opportunity cost" is used to describe the wasted months or years, the career progress foregone, the time and effort spent building a practice from which you will not achieve an adequate return.

Finally, there is the *emotional cost*, often considerable, of failing.

Most of us are accustomed to succeeding; admitting failure and starting over takes a toll on us and those close to us.

Making such a far-reaching mistake is particularly difficult for physicians to accept. Not only are we accustomed to getting what we want, but we believe we have a certain entitlement—rightly or wrongly—to compensation for the years invested, the sleep lost, the other sacrifices made during training. The acute disappointment of a failed practice then hits us just when we thought we were to be rewarded for our efforts. Such a situation need not occur if we just take the time and energy to choose a practice with care and attention.

Hard Costs

Before we examine the cost of changing jobs, let us look briefly at your financial status before you even begin to practice. The typical physician has accrued a staggering medical school debt. During the 1980s the figure ranged just under $50,000, and in many cases it was $70,000 plus. Moving into the 1990s the figures seem to be climbing even higher.

If you had sought traditional employment after college during this period rather than attending medical school and doing a residency, you might have started at an annual salary of $25,000 and progressed to $50,000 or $60,000 in those years, earning a total of perhaps $350,000 over that period. Instead, let us say that you earned roughly $100,000 during residency.

Add your debt to this sum, plus the possible but foregone return on investments, and it is easily seen that you must out-earn your age peers by more than $350,000 before you are merely even with them in terms of dollars. Only then can you start reaping the financial rewards from the additional investment in your education.

It is apparent that most of us start out in considerable debt, leery about adding to that financial burden. It is a fact of life, however, that by opening a practice or even taking a job we are forced to incur substantial financial risk. A good illustration is the story of Michelle, the physician who sadly decided to work at a walk-in clinic to distance herself from the intensity of her training program.

Despite the fact that the cost to her to set up a practice was minimal (as an employee of an established concern), it amounted to the following: state medical license fee $500; county medical society dues $150; state medical society dues $150; legal advice $1500; accounting services $2000; professional stationery $300; malpractice liability insurance $5000.

Michelle, though, soon left the clinic for an HMO. Although her new employment was only about forty miles away, it was in a neighboring state. Michelle then faced membership fees in the new county and state medical societies and had to duplicate nearly all the other expenditures as well. Her legal fees were nearly twice as much the second time around, because the HMO contract was twice as long and as complicated as the brief document used by the walk-in clinic. She also had moving costs, which amounted to just under $4500.

She had bought a house and had a difficult time selling it; hence she was making mortgage payments of $1500 a month while at the same time paying $600 a month to rent an apartment at her new location. She was still smarting from the loss of approximately $3000 in the "closing" costs on her first home (loan origination fee, title search, legal fees). There was a matching set of costs on the other end as well when she decided to sell the house; this time it was realtor's commission, termite inspection, advertising expenses, and of course the ubiquitous legal fees. That total tab came close to $9000. The worst news came just when Michelle thought she had come to grips with everything: It was spelled t-a-i-l. When you leave a practice these days, you may have to purchase tail coverage for your malpractice insurance. Michelle was blind-sided. She had not required her employer to provide such coverage; in fact she had never heard of it.

TAIL COVERAGE

As recently as the early 1980s, physicians usually bought "occurrence"-type liability insurance. Such policies covered physicians for losses arising from their professional activity during the policy period (e.g., for the year 1975) even if a lawsuit was filed many years later. If a physician made a clinical error in 1975 but was not sued until 1979, his occurrence policy covered the damage award—up to the policy limits, of course.

Today there are few malpractice insurance carriers willing to provide occurrence coverage. Instead, they offer "claims made" coverage, which covers only claims filed or incidents reported *while the policy is in force.* There is no coverage for claims filed after the policy expires, even if the alleged mistake occurred during the time the policy was in effect.

At the clinic, Michelle bought claims-made liability insurance from XYZ carrier on January 1, 1988, which became her "retroactive" date. The policy covered her from that date until the end of the policy period, coinciding in this case with the end of the calendar year. The presumption was that she would renew the policy year after year, thereby covering herself always back to her "retro" date. Therefore if someone sued her in 1990 for a 1988 incident, the policy in effect in 1990 would cover her because it represents a continuation, in effect, of the policy initiated in 1988.

Michelle left the clinic after just a year, however, and her new employer bought its malpractice coverage from another carrier, not the XYZ insurance company. Michelle then was forced to buy an extension of her first policy—"tail insurance"—from XYZ to protect her from future claims. Typically, such extended coverage costs close to 150% of the first year's premium. It is obvious why claims made insurance has become an effective deterrent to switching practices, even for the most unhappy physician.

Martin, the obstetrician who walked blindly into the New England community that had just had a bad experience with another male obstetrician, is an even more vivid example of the financial risk of starting a practice. The community had agreed to lease office space for Martin during his first year. Outfitting costs were his, however, which included furnishing three examination rooms, a private office/ consultation room, a nurse's station, and a waiting room. In addition, he set up a business office complete with telephone, computer, desks, chairs, file cabinets, stationary, and a complete set of color-coded medical records. He bought simple machines to equip a modest laboratory and leased his ultrasound equipment. The project cost Martin over $100,000. On top of that, his insurance premiums came to about $45,000.

Practice start-up costs are situation- and specialty- specific. On the one extreme, hospital-based physicians (e.g. pathologists and anesthesiologists) and physicians joining an established group need little or nothing to get started. If they are not employees (which they often are), such physicians may need malpractice insurance, licensure and membership fees, and a billing arrangement. Even physicians who work as independent contractors for hospitals, groups, or staffing agencies often get malpractice insurance and billing services from the "sponsoring" organization.

At the other end of the spectrum are the office-based physicians— from the simple rural family practitioner to the sophisticated suburban orthopedic surgeon—who set up practice independently. These physicians require office space, furniture, medical and business equipment, stationery, supplies, and staff. When you consider that a good chair for a waiting room or business office costs close to $300, the price tag for basic "outfitting" can easily be $100,000 to $150,000. Sophisticated laboratory and radiographic equipment are extra. If a building is purchased, there are mortgage costs for the building and the land it is on; otherwise, there are lease payments for the required space.

The costs themselves are frightening, but it gets harrowing when you consider that income only dribbles in when you first open the doors of your practice. A steady stream is not seen for several months after the billing starts.

What happens if you must change your practice? When Martin, the New England obstetrician, left town, he needed money in a hurry to meet the obligations he had assumed. His answer was to join a group and accept a salary. He returned the equipment he had leased but was forced to pay a penalty to cancel the arrangement. The furniture and equipment he had purchased went into storage and he thus had an additional monthly expense. He finally sold it at an 80% loss to a physician getting started in another town. Finally, he had to pay for tail coverage.

These stories are not intended to horrify you, simply to make you aware of the possible financial consequences of choosing a practice poorly. Image how the costs could mount up if you change jobs in rapid succession.

Opportunity Costs

Job failure invariably sparks self-reflection, an attempt to place mistakes in perspective and take stock. Such reflection is healthy, but it often fails to acknowledge one of the obvious debits of a bad practice situation—the better use you could have made of that time.

Consider David, the anesthesiologist who joined a group that was locked in a struggle with the new hospital administrator. David was lucky in that he lingered no more than a year in that situation. Nevertheless, when he reflects on his experience, David focuses on the fact that he would have been a year closer to partnership in his new practice if he had not wasted time in the first one, as well as a year closer to vesting in his new pension and profit-sharing plan. He puts a dollar value on his loss of seniority in the new situation and the lost year of contributions to the previous practice's plan.

David can probably calculate the actual cost of moving to that first community, moving again, and buying and selling the house, but he can only estimate the indirect costs of making the change. Moreover, he knows that had those dollars—as well as the money he spent for tail coverage—gone into certificates of deposit, it would have amounted to a considerable sum by the time his children are ready for college.

The move was also costly for David's wife. She was a medical librarian in their previous location but could only find a job in the local public library in the second location. In addition to sustaining a significant pay cut, she is overqualified and underchallenged in her new situation. The difference between what she wound up earning and what she could have earned is indeed an opportunity cost.

So far we have discussed simple opportunity cost. There is yet another aspect to the concept of opportunity cost as it relates to a choice of medical practice: A poor choice may limit opportunities in the future. Think back to Duncan, who first left an HMO because he did not like the way it scrimped on care, and then quit another group because of measures the employer utilized to increase practice revenue.

Duncan now has a better sense of where he belongs in the physician job market, what he wants and needs from his medical employment. Unfortunately, he may find the market no longer so eager to take him in. It matters not that Duncan's only problem was his high ethical standards. He now has two black marks on his resume and two lukewarm references to "recommend" him. In every future interview he will have to overcome the suspicion that "there might be skeletons in the closet." The lack of enthusiastic support from former colleagues speaks volumes.

In the smaller, less populated specialties, e.g., neurosurgery or radiation oncology, this problem is far worse than in the larger specialties. The old-boy networks are obviously smaller and, in the extreme: "Everyone knows everyone knows everyone." If others are not saying good things about you, you may find your opportunities thin. In terms of the price of choosing a practice poorly, then, the cost includes a blemished resume.

Emotional Costs

When a physician chooses a practice poorly, resulting in an early departure and a fresh start elsewhere, there are more than bills to pay and opportunity costs to lament. Most likely, there is also a psyche to repair.

Almost by definition, doctors are ambitious. We set high goals for ourselves and work hard to achieve them. We bring great expectations to our first job, believing it will provide personal and professional satisfaction as intense as the commitment we brought to our professional preparation. There is little chance that an unhappy departure from a practice will come with no emotional damage.

Should it happen to you, in addition to the hurt, you may experience a loss of confidence. A major failure is something you have probably not experienced or even considered, and now you are dealing not with the mere idea of it but its reality. Even if the outcome was not your fault, it has probably created doubt in your mind about "fitting in," getting along.

You must also face the fact that it does not look good to job-hop. A short stopover on the resume often puts you on the defensive during subsequent job interviews. Whereas one false start is normally overlooked, two quick moves raise a question in almost every interviewer's mind, and three doubtless reduce the percentage of openings for which you will be seriously considered, depending on your tenure in each position and, of course, the "real" reasons for your departure.

The failed practice is a blow to your spouse and children too. Each family member has to deal with his own resulting problems. If the family moves, it means that the children experience a break in educational and social continuity. It means the end of neighborhood relationships, religious group activities, Little League, and club memberships—each taking an emotional toll. Both sets of (grand)-parents have to adjust their perspective, modifying their pride in "my (grand)son(in-law) the doctor."

Change itself creates stress, which generates its own set of problems for all those affected. For the sensitive doctor/spouse/parent there may be guilt as well: You chose the wrong practice, you failed to make a go of it, and now others must suffer.

A word of caution. In the wake of a bad experience with a person or a situation, there is a tendency to let the negative characteristics of that experience unduly influence the decision about the next person or situation because we tend to emphasize factors or features "to be avoided." It is best to balance this tendency with a clear understanding of what *is* wanted. For example, when a practice fires its business manager in part because he was loud and overbearing, chances are that the partners will look next for a person who is mild and accommodating. What the practice really requires is someone who is neither obnoxious nor passive, whose managerial style is assertive but pleasant.

When you focus on a single blade of grass, the rest of the world is out of focus; when you focus on one issue, other relevant ones may well receive inadequate consideration, especially when the issue is emotionally charged. Emerging from a failed practice, you are not in an ideal frame of mind for choosing your next practice; you will be paying the emotional price for many months to come.

Final Statement

The people described in this book entered the "real world" with credentials and recommendations that are probably as good as yours. One thing we learn from their stories is clear: As we near the end of training, we have a final, major career investment to make. We must devote considerable attention to choosing where and how we want to practice lest we inflict unnecessary hurt on ourselves and our family, and hamstring an otherwise promising career.

Know Yourself

Getting to know yourself is the first key step in choosing a practice wisely. You must have the clearest possible picture of who you are and what you want out of life: what turns you on and what puts you off; what you like to do and what you prefer to avoid doing; what makes you jump out of bed in the morning and what makes you want to roll over and go back to sleep.

Your goal should be to put a round peg (you) in a round hole (your future practice)—to create a "good fit" between what you need and want on one hand and the life circumstances you choose on the other. In this chapter we talk about "the peg" and how to define its shape as clearly and accurately as possible. In the next chapter we will talk about "the hole," the practice and community that will provide you a comfortable setting in which to work and live.

> "Cheshire-puss," she began, rather timidly—
> "Would you tell me which way I ought to go from here?"
> "That depends a good deal on where you want to get to," said the cat.
> "I don't much care where," said Alice.
> "Then it doesn't matter which way you go," said the cat.
>
> Lewis Carroll, *Alice in Wonderland*, Putnam Publishing, 1987

Goals drive the decision-making process, as decisions are effective only in terms of the ultimate purpose. Without goals, you cannot develop a sensible plan for getting from here to there. A course of action has little value per se; it is good or bad only in terms of what you are trying to accomplish. Therefore, when deciding where and how you want to practice, you must begin with your goals and work backward.

In the broadest terms, let us say your goals are professional success and personal happiness. Success and happiness come from getting what you want out of life, which, in turn, usually involves having work that suits you, that "fits" well with who you are and how you like to function.

Starting at that point and working backward, the first step in finding work that suits you is understanding who you are and how you like to function—your basic personality type. That understanding should steer you toward the *type* of work that suits you and that therefore will probably make you happy. Getting to know yourself also calls for clarifying and prioritizing your individual preferences. Having chosen medicine as a career, you must determine what you want from a medical position, the job attributes that would make you happy.

You must thus "examine" yourself on two levels: Level I designates "intrinsic" factors, the fundamentals of who you are and how you like to function. These factors—your basic personality type—are ingrained, fixed, and beyond your control. Level II refers to "extrinsic" factors: what you are looking for, both tangible and intangible, from your job and your non-professional pursuits. Level II factors are less deep-seated in your being than level I factors. They are the more transitory needs, wants, and desires—things that may be important to you at a given point but that are apt to change with time, circumstance, and experience.

Level I: Personality Type

In 1920 the psychoanalyst Carl Jung (disagreeing with Freud, Adler, Sullivan, and Fromm) emphasized that people are different in fundamental ways, even though they share instincts that motivate them.

One instinct is no more important than the other, said Jung. What is important is the "preference"* we exhibit for "how we function." Our preference for a given function is characteristic, and we can be typed by it. Thus Jung continued the tradition started by Hippocrates of describing people in terms of their temperament—their personality type.

The concept of temperament was later replaced by "dynamic psychology" on the one hand and "behaviorist psychology" on the other. The Jungian concept was revived during the 1950s, however, and has since been refined by Isabel Myers and Katheryn Briggs, who developed an instrument to "measure" personality: the Myers-Briggs Type Indicator (discussed in more detail later).

Your personality type, according to Jung and others, is inborn, ingrained, and therefore nearly immutable. Preferences for perceiving, doing, or thinking about things in certain ways may strengthen or weaken over time, but your basic personality type does not change. For example, an introvert can try to sell insurance, but the attempt to fit into the salesman's mold distorts his underlying form: Remove the fangs of a lion and behold a toothless lion, not a domestic cat.

This basic truth is applicable to all phases of life. An attempt to change your spouse, for example, may bring some alteration, but the result is probably more a scar than a transformation. People are what they are. A critical aspect of life is *appreciating and accepting people for who and what they are.*

In searching for a practice, there is a particularly good reason for determining your personality type. Getting a good fit between "who you are" on the one hand and the type of professional situation you choose on the other requires that you recognize the "you" involved. A "goodness of fit" with your professional setting is critical.

MYERS-BRIGGS TYPE INDICATOR

Your temperament, or personality type, can be characterized using the Myers-Briggs Type Indicator. This marvelous instrument is ex-

---

*Note that the word "preference" is used throughout this discussion and in later references to it as Jung used it, not in the usual sense of the word.

plained in more detail and available for self-administration in *Please Understand Me* (by David Keirsy and Marilyn Bates, Gnosology Books Ltd., Del Mar, CA, 1984) and in *Gifts Differing* (by Isabel Briggs Meyers with Peter Meyers, Consulting Psychologists Press, Inc., Palo Alto, CA, 1980), books from which I have borrowed liberally in this chapter and which I consider indispensable to self-analysis and therefore to the search for the perfect practice.

The Myers Briggs Type Indicator test (MBTI) is based on four pairs of characteristics, each pair designating an important dimension or aspect of one's personality: extroversion/introversion; sensation/intuition; thinking/feeling; perceiving/judging. Jung said that one can predict differences in people's behavior by the extent to which they "prefer" or choose one way of doing or being over another; in other words, the extent to which they can be aptly characterized by one or the other of the traits in each of the four pairs developed by Jung and used in the MBTI.

As we explore the four dimensions of personality, keep in mind that Jung did not say that a person is either one or the other of the types. Rather, each of us can be extroverted in some areas and introverted in others, thinking as well as feeling and so on.

Extroversion/Introversion

The person who chooses people as a source of energy is probably extroverted, whereas the person who requires solitude to recover energy tends toward introversion. Extroverts, with a need for sociability, appear to be energized by interacting (talking, playing, working) with others. Extroverts experience loneliness when they are not in contact with people. The extreme extrovert may leave a party at 2:00 a.m. and be ready to go to another. His batteries are almost overcharged, having received so much energy from the interaction.

The introvert, on the other hand, is territorial; he desires space: private places in the mind as well as environmentally. Introverts draw energy from pursuing solitary activities, working quietly alone, reading, meditating, participating in activities that involve few or no other people. The extreme introvert may go to a party and after a half hour be ready to go home. Introverts are also likely to experience a sense of loneliness in a crowd. They report being most "alone," with a deep sense of isolation and disconnectedness, when surrounded by people.

It is not that introverts do not like to be around people; it simply drains their energy. Introverts need to find quiet places and solitary activities to recharge, whereas these activities exhaust the extrovert. Many introverts go through their lives believing that they should want more sociability and because of these guilty feelings do not provide adequately for their legitimate desire for territoriality, for breathing room. By contrast, if the extrovert must do research in a library he may have to exercise great will power to prevent himself, after fifteen minutes or so, from taking a "short brain break" and striking up a conversation with the librarian.

The question arises, "Does not an extrovert also have an introverted side and vice versa?" Yes. The preferred attitude, however—extroversion or introversion—is the one presented to the public, and the other side is "suppressed." The preferred attitude is thus expressed in the conscious personality.

Intuition/Sensation

The person who has a natural preference for sensation probably describes himself as "practical." Conversely, the person with a natural preference for intuition probably describes himself as "innovative."

Although extroversion and introversion are important concepts to grasp so we can understand ourselves and others, especially those with whom we live or work, they are minor preferences compared to the intuition/sensation duality. Of all the preferences, these two comprise the most important source of miscommunication, misunderstanding, and denigration. The results of these different approaches to viewing issues produces the widest gulf between people.

The "sensing" person wants, trusts, and remembers facts. He believes in experience and "knows" through experience (history), both personal and global. He might be described as earth-bound, grounded firmly in reality. When the "sensing" person talks to people, he is interested in their experience, their past. For example, when a sensation-preferring employer interviews someone for placement, he wants to know the applicant's experience—such information provides the interviewer with something he can understand, a sound basis for deciding whether to employ the applicant.

The intuition-preferring employer, on the other hand, has confidence not in what the applicant has done in the past but in what he verbalizes about the future of the organization—what he would do in a hypothesized situation, his vision of the possibilities for growth.

The sensation types (hereafter referred to as the "sensibles") take note of the actual and want to deal with that. They focus on what happened, rather than considering the future. These people remain in the "real world"; and when work is the issue, they tolerate no nonsense. The sensible observes details, his eyes tend to pick up on specific elements about the environment. The intuitive, on the other hand, scans or glances at things and people, aware only of what is related to his current preoccupation, thereby missing details.

The language that inspires the intuitive has no effect on the sensible. The intuitive finds appeal in metaphor and enjoys vivid imagery. He may daydream, read poetry, enjoy fantasy and fiction. The possible is always in front of him, pulling on his imagination like a magnet. The future hólds an attraction for the intuitive; the past and today do not. Because his head is often in another world, the intuitive can be subject to greater error about facts than the sensible, who pays more attention to what is going on about him.

For the intuitive, life is around the bend, on the other side of the mountain, just beyond the curve of the horizon. He can speculate for hours about possibilities. He sometimes finds complex ideas coming to him as a complete whole, unable to explain how he knew. These visions, intuitions, or hunches may show up in any realm—technology, sciences, mathematics, philosophy, the arts, or one's social life.

Of course, sensibles also have hunches, but they pay little attention to them; and after several years of ignoring their intuitions, not acting on them, not trusting them, the intuition is heard as mere static. The penalty one pays for ignoring that inner voice is that it diminishes. The penalty paid by those who prefer imagination—the intuitives—is that if they ignore reality too long they may end up out of touch with their environment.

The intuitive lives in anticipation. Whatever *is* can be better, or different, and today is seen as only a way station. Consequently, intuitives often experience a vague sense of dissatisfaction and rest-lessness. They are often bothered by reality, constantly looking to-ward possibilities of changing or improving the actual. The intuitive can skip from one activity to the next, completing none. Jung de-scribed the intuitive as one who seeds a field and then moves on to another project before the crop even breaks ground, looking for new fields to sow.

To the sensible, the intuitive appears flighty, impractical, and unre-alistic. The intuitive, on his part, views the sensible as plodding and exasperatingly slow to see possibilities for tomorrow.

Thinking/Feeling

People who prefer to make choices on an impersonal basis were called thinking types by Jung. People who prefer the personal ap-proach were called feeling types. Both of these ways of selecting what to do or not to do are necessary and useful. It is simply a matter of personal comfort. Some people are more comfortable with imper-sonal, objective judgments and uncomfortable with personal judg-ments. Others are more comfortable with value judgments and less comfortable with being objective and logical. Extreme feeling types are uncomfortable with rule-governed choices and regard the act of being impersonal as almost inhuman. Dedicated thinking types, on the other hand, sometimes look on emotion-laden decisions and choices as muddle-headed. It is well to remember, though, that all of us are capable of both types of decision-making.

People who use the feeling preference as the basis for decisions may claim that the thinking people are "heartless, stony-hearted, or have ice in their veins"—that they are "cold, remote intellectualizers who are without the milk of human kindness." On the other hand, the thinking preference people, who base decisions on impersonal principles, may claim that the feeling people are "too soft hearted, unable to take a firm stand, incapable of standing up in the face of opposition"—that they are "emotional, illogical thinkers and intel-lectual dilettantes who wear their hearts on their sleeves."

People with the feeling preference may have a better chance than the "thinkers" of developing their other side, as formal schooling addresses the thinking area far more than the feeling area. Unfortunately, the "thinkers" do not have an equal opportunity to develop their feeling side, which may remain relatively primitive.

Feeling types are sometimes seen as more emotionally sensitive than thinking types, but this is not the case. Both types can react emotionally with the same intensity; the feeling type, however, tends to make his emotional reactions more visible, so others view him as warmer and capable of deeper feelings than the thinking type.

When the feeling type becomes emotional, his hands become moist, color flushes or drains from his face, his body trembles, his heart beats faster. It is no wonder that others are affected by his reaction. Indeed, the emotional reactions of such people tend to be contagious and to generate heat.

In contrast, when the thinking type becomes emotional, the same body reactions are not as evident and therefore not as much noticed by others. Thus thinking people are often described as cold and unemotional, whereas in reality they may be experiencing intense emotion. The thinking person, in fact, is sometimes embarrassed by a show of intense emotions, whereas the feeling person may enjoy an excessive show of feelings.

The thinking and feeling preferences need not cause serious problems in interpersonal relations if the two ways of going about making decisions are understood and appreciated. As with the other preferences, these two types can complement each other rather advantageously. Once the feeling person understands that the thinking person does indeed have deep, though not always visible emotions, and once the thinking person recognizes that the feeling person can think logically, though it may not always be verbalized, misunderstandings between them are apt not to arise.

Judging/Perceiving

The key difference between judging and perceiving types boils down to the question: Do I prefer to get closure and settle things, or do I prefer to keep options open and fluid?

Persons who choose closure over open options are likely to be the judging type, whereas those who prefer to keep things open and fluid are probably the perceiving type. The "judger" is apt to experience a sense of urgency until a pending decision is made. The perceiving person, in contrast, is more apt to resist making the decision, wishing that more data could be accumulated. As a result, when the perceiving person finally makes a decision he may still have a feeling of uneasiness and restlessness, whereas the judging person in the same situation may have feelings of relief and satisfaction.

Judgers tend to establish deadlines and take them seriously, expecting others to do the same. Perceivers tend more to look at deadlines as alarm clocks, almost as if the deadline were used more as a signal to start than to complete a project. This preference can be a source of irritation in relationships because judgers push for a decision whereas perceivers hold out for additional data and perhaps more options.

Apparently, all judging people—whether intuitive or sensible, thinking or feeling, introverted or extroverted—share an attitude toward work and play that is different from the attitude of the perceivers. The judging types seem to believe that work comes before all else, an outlook that has a marked effect on what they are willing to do to get the job done (including perhaps preparation, maintenance, and clean-up afterward). Perceivers, on the other hand—whether intuitive or sensible, thinking or feeling, introverted or extroverted—seem to have a play ethic. They are far more playful and less serious than the judging types. If the process of work is not directly instrumental (is simply preparation, maintenance, or clean-up), the perceiver may balk at doing it or will find something else to do. Perceivers are much more insistent than the judgers that the work process be enjoyable. It might be said that perceivers are process-oriented, whereas judgers are outcome-oriented.

These two types tend to criticize each other, especially at work. Judging people have been heard to describe perceivers as "indecisive," "procrastinating," "aimless," "resistive," and "critical." Perceivers have become impatient with judgers because they feel pressured and hurried by what they view as unnecessary urgency and an unfortunate tendency to "jump to conclusions." Perceivers occasionally claim that judgers make hasty decisions and are "driven," "too task oriented," "pressured and pressuring," "rigid and inflexible," and "arbitrary." Usually, irritation by another's preference dissipates when these behaviors are studied and understood. With continued understanding, most people even become fascinated and entertained by these differences and find ways to make allowances for another person's way.

Temperament

The above section describes fundamental ways in which people differ. Under the theory we have been considering, people create their "type" through exercise of their individual preferences—the way they prefer to use their minds in becoming aware of things, people, occurrences, and ideas (perception), and in coming to conclusions about what they have perceived (judgment). The interests, values, needs, and habits of mind that naturally result from any set of preferences tend to produce a recognizable set of traits and potentialities, which we have been referring to as "personality."

Individuals can, therefore, be described in part by stating their four preferences, such as extroverted/intuitive/thinking/perceiving (ENTP) or introverted/intuitive/feeling/judging (INFJ). An "ENTP" or "INFJ" can be expected to be different from others in ways characteristic of his type. The Myers-Briggs Type Indicator categorizes people into one of sixteen such personality types and describes in detail the traits to be expected from people whose personality is structured by the four preferences that make up that type. It is beyond the scope of this book to portray each of the possible sixteen personality types. Instead, the four fundamental temperaments that underlie these sixteen personality types are described, including how the interests, values, and needs of such people may fit into various professional settings.

As used here, *temperament* denotes a moderation or unification of otherwise disparate forces, a tempering of opposite influences, an overall coloration or tuning, a thematization of the whole, a uniformity of the diverse. Your temperament is that which places a signature or thumbprint on your actions, making it recognizably yours.

There are four recognized temperament types, as indicated by Hippocrates centuries ago and by Spranger more recently: Promethean, Apollonian, Dionysian, Epimethian. These types are convenient for predicting and explaining behavior and form the "core" of the sixteen personality types that evolve from the MBTI. Let us look at each of these temperament types to see how much they can tell us about the type of work we are best suited for and how to position ourselves properly in the medical world.

Promethean Temperament

Prometheus gave man fire, the symbol of light and energy, to make him more like the gods. By harnessing light and energy, mankind has gained control and understanding of nature. To understand and control nature is to possess power, and it is the desire for that power that sets the Promethean apart from others.

> Power fascinates this type of person. Not power over people, but power over nature: To be able to understand, control, predict, and explain realities. Note that these are the four aims of science: control and understanding, prediction and explanation. Scratch a Promethean, find a scientist.
>
> These forms of power, however, are but means to an end, one best expressed by the word *competence*. So it's not exactly power that the Promethean wants, but rather competencies, capabilities, abilities, capacities, skills, ingenuity—the repertoire.
>
> The Promethean loves intelligence, which means doing things well under varying circumstances. In the extreme, he can even be seen as addicted to acquiring intelligence, hooked on storing up wisdom, just as Aesop's ant must store up goodies.*

It takes little imagination to visualize this type of person coming into his own in academia. His inclination to be the scientist fits well with the research and publication requirements of academic positions; teaching, challenging others and being challenged could be viewed as appropriate to the person constantly driven to improve his competence, control, mastery, and understanding of the world around him.

On rounds, for example, the Promethean faculty member would absolutely delight in displaying his storehouse of knowledge and wisdom, and in the operating room would find it especially satisfying to be able to demonstrate his surgical skills to an appreciative audience of residents and students.

---

*David Keirsey and Marilyn Bates, *Please Understand Me*, Gnosology Books Ltd., Del Mar, CA, 1984, pp 47–48.

Apollonian Temperament

People driven to pursue extraordinary goals, prominent among them self-fulfillment, are said to have an Apollonian temperament.

> The Apollonian hungers for self-actualization, to be what he's meant to be and to have an identity that's uniquely his. His endless search causes him guilt, believing that his real self is somehow less than it ought to be. To be lost in the crowd, to have the same meaning as others, to share a faceless identity is to not be at all. Only a life of significance, making a difference in the world, will satisfy his hunger for unique identity.
>
> In order to make a difference and to maintain individuality, the unique contributions made by the Apollonian personality must be recognized. No matter how this type of person structures his time and relationships, he needs to have *meaning*. He wants his importance appreciated or, at the very least, recognized. Only through this kind of feedback does the Apollonian know he has unique identity.
>
> Apollonians as a group show little interest in buying or selling or any commercial occupations, nor do they find the physical sciences particularly attractive. The prefer to work with words, and need and want to be directly or indirectly in communication with people.*

Can you imagine an Apollonian personality sequestered away in a small laboratory doing bench research? It would be just as difficult to imagine him putting in his eight hours as a faceless cog at an HMO or working at a walk-in clinic housed in a neighborhood shopping center. Only an Apollonian with no basic understanding of "who he is and how he likes to function" would consider that type of work. Such individuals would probably do best as missionaries, prominent practitioners in smaller communities, or leaders of medical groups, hospitals, or organizations doing "important" work.

Dionysian and Epimethian Temperament

The final examples of personality types are the Dionysian and the Epimethian temperaments, a study in contrasts.

---

*David Keirsey and Marilyn Bates, *Please Understand Me*, Gnosology Books Ltd., Del Mar, CA, 1984, pp 57–63.

For the Dionysian, the bottom line is *freedom*. He won't be tied or bound, confined or obligated. To be independent, to do as he wishes when he wishes, that's the ideal. He has a play ethic. The Epimethian, on the other hand, is compelled to be bound and obligated. He defines himself by his responsibilities, and thus he needs them. His is a work ethic.

This is not to say the Dionysian doesn't acquire goals and ties, just as the rest of us do. He does, of course, but they're fewer and more tentatively held. If the ties become too numerous or too binding, the Dionysian will grow restless and soon be gone. In him, restrictions of any sort tend to spark an urge to take off.

By contrast, the Epimethian must *belong*. With that, he carries a sense of obligation, duty and responsibility. Supporting his sense of responsibility is a desire for hierarchy. For the Epimethian, the hierarchical structure of society is the essence of society. There should be subordinance and superordinance. There should be rules to govern the interaction of people (the members of society), certainly in the city, schools, church, and corporation. And one's status in such social units must be earned—one must do his part.

The Dionysian supports his fraternal and libertarian outlook with a belief in, and desire for, equality. One is equal to others in whatever social unit one belongs to, and status at any level is a matter of luck or happenstance. As a student, he'd view the professor not as a superior person, but as just another man, an equal, who happens to be filling the "professor" slot at the moment.

And rules? Why those are merely disguised means of maintaining the status-quo one acquired by accident.*

It is difficult to imagine the Dionysian in a military or government job or in a Veterans Administration hospital setting which would be likely to please the Epimethian. In contrast, try to imagine the Epimethian doing locum tenens, traveling from one practice to the next with blocks of free time in between—a job that is tailor made for the Dionysian. The Dionysian would have difficulty in a large multi-specialty group, with a structured, hierarchical chain of command, rigorous peer review, and heavy-handed requirements for conformity in practice style. The Epimethian, however, would be happiest in

---

*David Keirsey and Marilyn Bates, *Please Understand Me*, Gnosology Books Ltd., Del Mar, CA, 1984, pp 31–47.

precisely that sort of environment; a small, freewheeling group of colleagues would make him decidedly uncomfortable.

VALUE OF LEVEL I INTROSPECTION

Self-analysis can give you a sense of the *type* of work that is likely to resonate best with your fundamental temperament or personality. Level I analysis is important because personality type is firmly established, and you are not, as some people like to believe, infinitely adaptable to the circumstances of one or another professional situation.

Knowing your personality type gives you a better sense of the kind of activities, pursuits, and involvements you are likely to find stimulating, satisfying, fulfilling—or disagreeable, disruptive, incompatible. Although having this knowledge does not guarantee you the perfect practice, not knowing it may well doom you to an entirely unsuitable one.

How then do you determine your personality type? Career counselors can test you in countless and detailed ways. I rely greatly on the Myers-Briggs Type Indicator because it is relatively simple, inexpensive, and widely accepted as state-of-the-art. As a health professional, you can easily secure and self-administer this test, or you can even use its short form, which is available in Kersey and Bates's *Please Understand Me.*

By following the suggestions offered above, you should wind up with a personality self-portrait that fits well and gives you a good idea of your values, needs, and preferences and directs you toward the type of work for which you are best suited.

Level II: External Factors

Level I exploration has clarified your personality type. The next step in better understanding yourself is to delineate your "external" wants and needs.

What would it take to make you happy? Is money important to you? Power? Prestige? Free time? Clean air? Good schools? Availability of museums? Wide open spaces? Doubtless, you have a combination of wants. Because happiness is the general goal we started off with and getting what you want should move you closer to that goal, defining and prioritizing your wants is an important step toward happiness.

For the purpose of considering "external" needs, it is convenient to group them into categories. "Personal" and "professional" desires are major categories each of which can be broken down into two smaller subcategories: "tangible" factors (e.g., money) and "intangible" factors (e.g., prestige).

Thinking in terms of categories allows you to enumerate and prioritize what you want within each category and then to consider the balance or tradeoffs between categories. The question of balance is tricky. Simply put, our lives normally require a balance, or resonance, between the personal and the professional and between the tangible and the intangible. Ideally, you will meet the demands of your professional role as you find personal satisfaction; and as you attain the intangible satisfactions of life, you will also find yourself warm, dry, and well fed.

Unfortunately, it is not always that simple. Although you seek a balance between the personal and professional dimensions of your life, you often find the two competing. Thus an important part of knowing yourself is knowing where the balance point lies for you.

On level I, you deal with such questions as "Do you live to work or work to live?" On level II you deal with issues such as money versus time off, better insurance versus more funding for your pension plan, more time for research versus time for teaching or seeing patients.

Although there is no shortcut to finding where the balance point lies between competing needs or interests, the suggestions in this chapter should help considerably. Organizing your wants and needs into logical categories coupled with honest self-appraisal should help you understand and balance them. The process of sorting considerations into the major categories "personal" (what you want and need for yourself as a person or for your family) and "professional" (what you want and need in your role as a physician) as suggested above, is rather straightforward and requires little explanation. Dealing effectively with the tangible and intangible subcategories is more challenging. Therefore, the rest of this chapter is devoted primarily to those subcategories. The chapter concludes by highlighting some key considerations in the personal sphere, considerations that might fall between the floorboards because of a myopic focus on only professional issues.

INTANGIBLE NEEDS

The psychological needs and longings that you bring to your various roles in life are intangible but real. Here the boundary between intrinsic (level I) and extrinsic (level II) needs becomes hazy because your personality portrait is characterized in part by the extent of your longing for power, position, self-actualization. Although no less real than a paycheck, your psychological needs are often more elusive and difficult to define. Nevertheless, they are key determinants of your happiness, and you cannot afford to overlook or fail to assess them.

Achievement

Achievement is an important intangible factor. Physicians are generally high-achievement people compared with the general population, but within the medical ranks some are more achievement-oriented than others.

- Would you be happy in a low-profile practice?
- Is it your ambition to bring modern medicine to a Third World country?
- Do you dream of discovering the cure for cancer and winning the Nobel Prize?

To determine what achievement means to you, think about your attitude toward achievement.

- Do you see achievement as an individual accomplishment, or do you view it in organizational terms?

If achievement is an individual concept for you and you have the requisite aptitude for research, the laboratory might be the place for you. In contrast, if achievement is an organizational matter to you and you have the mind and temperament for management, perhaps you should aspire to be the managing partner of a large group.

Achievement may simply mean financial security—living in a fancy home, driving a luxury car, or sending your children to expensive schools. If so, and the practice of medicine is your means to those ends, greater weight should be placed on other factors, probably the "tangibles," when determining what you want from your practice. Whatever your attitudes and choices, the important thing is to translate vague, generalized concepts into specific, functional ideas that you can more readily understand and with which you can work.

Success

Another intangible factor is the concept of success. As with achievement, it is important to move from the generality of the idea to an operational definition of what it means to you.

• To what extent is your personal "success" a matter of matching your accomplishments with those of your colleagues?
• Or are you content with self-satisfaction?
• If you are highly competitive, can you handle losing? Must you be number one, or can you accept being second best?

If the answer to the last question is "no," it is fairly important that you choose a professional pond in which you are likely to be the biggest fish.

Competence

Competence, another intangible factor, is not something we usually regard as a need.

• To what extent do you define success by your level of proficiency?
• Does your quest for competence override such issues as where you work and with whom?

If maximum proficiency is important, you probably should look for a situation that gives you the greatest number of referrals in your area of special expertise, allows you to perform the most procedures, or maximizes your time in the operating room.

Autonomy/Power

Think about your need for autonomy and power.

- How important is it for you to influence or direct others?
- How good are you at wielding such influence?
- Must you be master of your fate, or can you accept direction from others?
- To what extent do you need a powerful person above you in order to feel secure in a situation?

One way to address these and other questions associated with your assessment of "external" factors is to use a "retrospectoscope." Reflect on your past dealings and interactions. During residency, for example:

- How did you relate to the program director?
- Did you bristle at orders and directives, or feel relieved when they were finally made clear?
- How did you interact with nurses, ward clerks, secretaries?
- Were you good at giving orders, or did you come down with a case of sweaty palms when you had to push for a laboratory result or a transcription you had dictated days before?

A mismatch with respect to the need for and availability of autonomy, especially in the professional sphere, is a major source of dissatisfaction in medical practice. Therefore, when evaluating an opportunity, make sure you understand not only your own need for influence and autonomy but also who has what kind of authority in the practice. Where is the focus of power? Does it lie with physicians or with nonphysicians? Is it highly concentrated or well distributed? These and similar questions should give you a good idea of how much professional autonomy and control you are likely to attain in a given situation.

Prestige/Recognition

Prestige and recognition take many forms. Two extremes of medical practice are (1) being a small-town doctor and (2) holding a position in an academic referral center. The successful small-town physician is rewarded by patient adulation, whereas the academic has strong peer recognition. In a small town, the ubiquitous and friendly "Hi, doc, how are you?" from admiring townsfolk is heartwarming. On the other hand, publishing a paper in the *New England Journal of Medicine* would go virtually unnoticed in that community. In a large academic center the opposite is true. You are apt to be acknowledged by your colleagues for being published in the *Journal*, but you may go unacknowledged in the crowded hospital cafeteria.

The issue, then, is not only one of more or less prestige and recognition; it is how the prestige and recognition are manifested. How essential is it to you to hear a colleague say, "Hey, good job" or "Neat idea" or "That was good thinking. I was stumped, but you cleared it up for me"?

If prestige without peer acknowledgment is enough, you might be happy in a small town. However, if it takes collegial recognition to warm your soul, you might favor a position in a large group or other medical organization.

Freedom/Security

In our profession, as in much of life, there tends to be a tradeoff between freedom and security. To gain more of one, you often must sacrifice a measure of the other.

In a solo practice, for example, you are more or less free to do as you please, but you forego the established patient population, the predictable paycheck, and the coverage provided during time off that comes with a well established group practice. If you practice in a loose association with two or three colleagues who only share expenses, each of you may be able to practice without having to reconcile your activities with the expectations of your associates. In a large group, you may be required to practice according to guidelines that strongly influence all the members' clinical activities and decisions.

TANGIBLE NEEDS

Financial Attitudes

For many of us, the most important tangible need is money. In thinking about money, it makes sense to focus not on how much you can make but on how much is enough for you.

One way to arrive at a reasonable figure for how much is enough is to define the salary that would provide what you (realistically) want, at least for the near future. With this figure in mind, then, ask yourself if $5000 (1989 dollars) more would make a real change in your life. Would you live differently, do important things you could not do with less money? If so, your first figure was not high enough. What about an additional $10,000 or $25,000?

Everyone is familiar with the saying "You can't be too rich or too thin." In truth, the unfettered drive for either goal can be counterproductive, if not pathological. Consider instead what the economists refer to as "the declining utility of each additional increment of income," also known as "marginal benefit." An income jump from $35,000 to $50,000 represents a meaninfgul increase in purchasing power and would likely improve your style of living. In contrast, if your income went from $300,000 to $315,000—the same absolute increase of $15,000—you probably would not notice the difference.

The point is that beyond a certain level of income other things, including the time and freedom to enjoy your life, usually become far more important than the additional money. Understanding that point helps put the money issue in perspective and, hopefully, will help you achieve a balance between money and other important considerations.

Keeping the "declining utility" concept in mind, let us reconsider the money issue.

- How much money do you need to live where and in the style you find comfortable?
- Taking into account the amount of money you know you need for basics, what will another $5000, $10,000, or $20,000 do for you?
- How important are the things the extra income will provide?

• Does their importance compare favorably with the importance of what you may have to sacrifice to earn that income—perhaps in terms of the extra time you might have had for teaching, for your family, or for personal pursuits?

Keep in mind, too, that there is a significant philosophical and psychological difference between pursuing money as an end in itself and making money as a "by-product" of pursuing something you find pleasure in doing. The heart surgeon who becomes wealthy because he derives great satisfaction from his surgery and its results is quite different from the surgeon who spends much of his time in the operating room because it is the most efficient way to expand his bank account. A variation of this theme is found in business, where it is not uncommon for the entrepreneur to view income as a way of "keeping score." To the idealistic entrepreneur, income is important not for what it does to his bank account but, rather, for what it reflects about the value of the product or service he provided and the effectiveness with which he did so.

Free Time

Considering that time is money, time can be viewed in economic terms, which means that free time is another important tangible need. As medicine becomes more a job and less a calling, we are increasingly disinclined to view ourselves as medical machines designed to run 24 hours a day, 52 weeks a year. For better or worse, that changing attitude encourages us to look more toward nonprofessional pursuits for happiness and fulfillment.

• To what extent do you find fulfillment outside of medicine and therefore need to be away from your job to pursue other endeavors?
• To what extent must the location of your medical practice accommodate your nonmedical activities?

Allowing adequate time away from your practice is important because, as discussed earlier, a life based solely on professional pursuits and achievements rests on a shaky foundation.

Work Environment

We all respond to our physical surroundings, often to an extent to which we are unaware. An environment that does not suit you may make you unhappy without your recognizing the problem. Therefore be sure to think about the suitability of the physical space in which you plan to work.

• Will you be satisfied with a cubicle where you can do your paperwork, or is it important for you emotionally to work in a handsome, well appointed office that elevates you psychologically and reminds you and those around you of your station in life?
• Can you work comfortably in a dingy government hospital, or do you feel better walking down carpeted halls with pictures hung on the wall?

Special Medical Interests

During the postgraduate years, we may pursue additional knowledge or training for reasons of intellectual stimulation, the need for technical mastery, or the prestige or advancement such pursuits might provide. We may give little thought to the marketability of the additional skills we acquire and therefore the likelihood of practicing or earning additional income from what we learn.

• What are your special medical interests?
• If you want to do research, how much time will be available for it? How much laboratory space? To what extent will you have to generate your own funding?
• If you enjoy surgery, what is the surgical case load likely to be?
• If you trained for several years in a subspecialty discipline, to what extent will you be able to practice in that area? Will limiting your practice to that subspecialty enhance your income, or cause financial hardship?

If you cannot be assured of the time you hoped for to pursue your special interests, or if such pursuits mean financial sacrifices, how will it affect you? Will you be devastated or mildly disappointed?

A Final Word on Tangibles and Intangibles

Happiness comes from satisfying a complex configuration of needs and desires. By getting to know yourself better, you come to understand the extent to which each factor—each need, interest, preference, goal—is important to you.

Our tangible needs tend to crowd out thoughts of intangible needs as we search for the elusive perfect practice. Care must be exercised not to underrate the importance of those intangible factors, however. Although they are the attitudes least easily identified (or faced), they are the very factors likely to support or undermine your choice of practice in the long run. In a high income profession such as medicine, the tangible needs tend to take care of themselves sooner or later, leaving you to consider if the important intangible needs associated with fulfillment and self-esteem have been satisfied. If these intangible needs have not been met, you will likely be unhappy, regardless of the tangible assets you have accumulated. (If you question this reasoning, examine Henry's case in Chapter 1!)

Personal Needs

Personal considerations of great importance are often overlooked when searching for a practice. This is not surprising as you have probably focused on professional considerations for most of your adult life and are still doing so, pushing other issues to the periphery by necessity.

Family Considerations

Family issues are generally among the most important personal issues in our lives. We usually seek frequent contact with our nuclear and extended families, and these family members exert a profound influence on us. The nature and location of a practice should reflect and accommodate family considerations.

Family influences are far-ranging:

- Your spouse's expectations
- Your baby's demands
- Your need to outdo your father

- Your older brother's financial problems
- Your younger sister's need for guidance
- Your parent's need to be taken care of
- Your determination to make your parents proud of you

Often the most compelling family considerations center around the needs and wants of your spouse.

- To what extent does satisfying your spouse preoccupy you?
- Can she or he be satisfied in the location you are contemplating?
- How will the demands placed on you by your practice mesh with the demands of your spouse? What tradeoff will you have to make to accommodate both?
- Does your spouse have education or career considerations that you must take into account, at least at some point?
- Do your spouse's activities require your involvement?

Interacting with children is another key consideration.

- Is it enough for you to tuck your children into bed after 20 minutes of "quality time," or do you want heavy involvement with them at least three full evenings a week plus weekends?
- Does the thought of "missing your kids growing up" plague you— or not concern you?
- Are family vacations the focal point of your life or a distraction from the more important business of your career?

Make a concerted effort to understand the role of your family in your life. Define how family considerations may limit you and, conversely, how they may expand and enrich you. How supportive and helpful are your family members? How demanding?

There are no right and wrong answers to such questions. However, if you fail to be honest and accurate, you are fooling only yourself. It is also well to remember that in addition to pleasing those around you, you must satisfy yourself as well. Anything less leads to trouble.

Personal Satisfaction

To abdicate your nonprofessional persona, to ignore your needs and interests apart from medicine, is to court disaster. "To thine own self be true" is applicable here. When choosing a practice, the wise physician takes into account personal interests and sources of satisfaction, and ensures that important personal pursuits—from the simple pleasures of backyard gardening to the excitement of attending major sports events or traveling to exotic places—can be accommodated.

- Do you want time for tennis? Is it enough for you to play on the town's two public courts, or do you need a court in your backyard?
- Are you willing to drive six hours to sail on a lake, or do you want to be within walking distance of an ocean marina?
- If you play the piano, must you have access to a concert caliber instrument, or can you be content to practice on a small upright in a spare room of your house?
- Do you fare well on food from the microwave, or must you have access to fine restaurants with extensive wine cellars?
- Do you like attending the ballet and opera, or can a decent television and stereo system satisfy your cultural desires?
- Is it enough to be within a two hour drive of a regional theater, or must you be within an easy cab ride of Broadway?

A practice that isolates you from personal activities of particular interest will produce a void you may find difficult or impossible to fill with satisfactions from the professional sphere alone.

Rules of the Road

Each of us is a complex person with many important roles and relationships. A good life/career decision is one that takes into account your specific needs and wants in regard to those roles and relationships. A balance is therefore sought. If too much weight is assigned to any one dimension of your life at the expense of others, in time it will probably pull you off track.

This chapter has been steering you toward self-exploration. To get the most from this process, you might consider the following key ground rules.

1. Keep your sights set on the ultimate purpose. Self-exploration is not an abstract exercise. It is essential that you know yourself so

you can clarify values and set goals. With this knowledge you can choose a practice that resonates with who you are and what you want out of life.

2. Be honest with yourself. Anything less than brutal candor borders on self-deception and boils down to a waste of time and energy.
3. Be explicit. Lay the facts on the table to be examined in the cold, clear light of day.

It is certainly acceptable if the results of your analysis are "for your eyes only," but to the extent that you can comfortably involve others do so. It is particularly important that "significant others" become involved at certain critical points, as they can help you be realistic and objective. They also can remind you, rightly so, that they too have a stake in your decisions.

Finding Out More About What You Want

Few would argue that getting in touch with who you are and what you want out of life is important. The above sections discussed ways to go about it. In addition to considering your needs and interests in terms of the categories described above, you can also benefit from thinking about the common denominators that underlie the activities you enjoy and the skills and talents you possess. Finally, a few last thoughts on setting goals may also help you chart a sensible course.

PREFERRED ACTIVITIES

Let us start with the activities you enjoy most. Your "retrospecto-scope" may help. Think back on courses taken, jobs held, activities engaged in, environments lived in. What about them pleased you or put you off? It is important to focus on these areas and come up with a clear picture of your likes and dislikes.

Perhaps you were a lifeguard once. Did you enjoy the adulation of the beach people or the morning solitude before anyone showed up? Maybe you were a pastry chef or a short-order cook. Did you like the dynamics of working in a kitchen, or did you merely tolerate the interaction with others because you liked watching your creations come out of the oven?

What hobbies have you pursued? Where do you go and what do you do on vacation? Given a free weekend, do you look for the liveliest party, whip up a gourmet feast for an intimate few, visit the museum, run off to the mountains, or sit by the fire with a good book?

You may also *fantasize* about and record what you would like to do given the right means and circumstances. Fickle though they may be, fantasies provide vital clues to what is important to you, and they shape your future more than you might realize. Remember, you do not have to share what you write down with anyone, so you can be honest.

When looking backward through your retrospectoscope or forward through your fantasies, look for *common denominators.*

- Were your most enjoyable experiences indoors or outdoors, competitive or cooperative, involving or excluding other people?
- Did they involve primarily the physical dimension or the spiritual?
- Was it the end result that pleased you most or the process of getting there?
- What was it about the process that was important or pleasing?

Identifying these threads, trends, and common denominators can help you recognize the *kinds* of things you like to do (as distinguished from specific activities) and the *kinds* of settings and circumstances you prefer (rather than a specific location or situation). The result will be a broader, more flexible view of yourself and the activities and environment most likely to make you happy. It will give you a solid base from which to examine the circumstances of each practice you look at.

For example, the list of the things you like to do may reveal that you like ocean racing, but the most important thing you discover from other items on the list is that being outdoors, on the water, in pursuit of adventure with the camaraderie of others are the key elements that underlie your interest in sailing. Does that mean that you must locate your practice where you can race sailboats? No, but it may well mean that you had better have access to that *type* of satisfaction. Perhaps you can substitute mountain climbing or whitewater kayaking for sailing adventures if you are offered an excellent professional opportunity in Wyoming.

Perhaps you like tennis—so much so that you want to play year round. What is it about tennis that you like so much? If it is the intense, competitive activity, you can find it in Minneapolis; you do not have to live in the sunbelt. Raquetball or squash, both indoor activities, can be substituted to meet your need for competition. If, on the other hand, you tolerate the competitive and aerobic requirements of tennis only because you like being outdoors, getting a tan, socializing, and sidling up to the country club bar, perhaps you should settle in a well-to-do suburban community in a warm, sunny climate.

It is now obvious that making lists is merely the first step, the next and more important step being the search for common denominators that underlie individual activities and endeavors. They are the signposts that can best guide you toward what is really important to you, the values and preferences that underlie your life choices.

SKILLS AND TALENTS

Your skills and talents represent another set of considerations when choosing where and how to practice. Definitions are in order here. A *skill* is acquired, something you have learned to do well. *Talent* is a broader concept; it is something you either have or do not have, a fundamental, innate ability. Mozart's musical talent was far beyond that of other musicians, some of whom, however, demonstrated nearly as much skill as Mozart on the keyboard.

Your skills and talents are assets, and it behooves you to identify them honestly and deploy them wisely. You can experience a great deal of satisfaction from situations that draw on your strengths and minimize your weaknesses, that allow you to develop your talent and use your skills to good advantage. Situations that do not provide these conditions can doom you to frustration and dissatisfaction, just like those that do not resonate with your personality.

As with the previous list-making exercises, patterns and common denominators help to highlight your skills and abilities. It is likely that you have relied on and applied them in past endeavors and have thought about using them in the future.

As before, it is important to ask for input from friends or family members who know you well. In fact, objective input is probably as important here as in any other aspect of the self-discovery process because your self-image may be somewhat idealized and therefore misleading. At least reconcile your beliefs and perceptions with the way others perceive you.

Goals can and often do change. Needs and wants may evolve. Your basic abilities, however, like your personality, are much less mutable. You cannot change the hand you are dealt; you can only play the cards more or less wisely.

GOALS

Finally, let us revisit the issue of goal setting. Formulating plans and strategies—whether in business, patient care, or life—requires that you start at the end and work backward.

The beauty of that approach lies in the fact that a firm, realistic objective itself begins to define what must be done to reach that end. That is, if you wish to reach Z, you must first arrive at Y; and to arrive at Y, you must first achieve X, and so on. The following simple example is a personal one.

> A teenage member of my family decided one spring that she wanted to visit Europe. The goal, then, was Europe. Having established the goal, we discussed what she had to do to get there. I pointed out that plane tickets were costly, and so if she wanted to go to Europe she had to acquire some money. We then began considering the jobs suitable for young ladies 15 years of age. Babysitting seemed to be the answer. We then thought about how she could get into the babysitting business. She elicited help from her mother to prepare a flyer advertising her services, which she then placed in mailboxes around the neighborhood.
>
> It was not long before the first requests came in, and within days her business was a successful venture. The bonus was that she learned a good deal about fundamental management issues: what to charge and how to convey her charges pleasantly but firmly to her customers. By the time the scheduled trip to Europe took place, she had made all the money she needed for the plane fare, and then some.

The message, of course, is that what began as a distant goal and daunting task became manageable and achievable by working backward from the objective one step at a time. When a task is approached in that way, the goal defines the actions you must take to reach that goal. Each step itself becomes a goal, something that must be achieved in order to approach the next step. It is similar to peeling an onion one layer at a time to get to its core. The most important elements in this process are following through tenaciously and learning as you go along.

With this type of goal setting, the more distant goals are characterized in more general terms than the closer, more clearly attainable objectives, which is as it should be. Circumstances and desires change over time, so it makes sense to allow some flexibility in your long-term goals and not to be overly specific. A "robust" formulation of where you want to be five, ten, or twenty years hence allows you to accommodate to the changes that inevitably occur over time.

What must be clear and specific is your next move or next series of moves. The football team marching down the field knows where the goal line is, but its focus is on the next first down. It keeps the goalpost in mind, but it recognizes that if it keeps making first downs it will surely wind up where it wants to be.

■ 4

Know the Job Market

There are over 500,000 physicians in the United States, and the nation's 127 medical schools graduate approximately 20,000 new ones each year. At the same time about 10,000 are lost to retirement, death, disillusionment, and the shoals of malpractice. Hence there is a net gain of about 10,000 physicians per year.

Doubtless you have heard of the "doctor glut." What a difference a decade makes. During the mid-1970s virtually every study on physician manpower reported that the country was short at least 50,000 physicians. Based on these figures the federal government undertook a massive manipulation of the medical marketplace by offering major incentives to increase the capacity of our medical schools and postgraduate training programs. The response was dramatic, and by the mid-1980s experts were forecasting an oversupply of 70,000 physicians by 1990, worsening to 145,000 by the end of the century. Physician overpopulation is expected to be especially severe in certain specialties and the fee-for-service segment of the profession.

The "market" for physician services, then, is evolving dramatically from a seller's to a buyer's market. If current trends in supply and forecasts of demand prove accurate, the potential impact on job-seeking physicians will be enormous.

Geographic Imbalance

That is the bad news. The good news is that physician supply and demand is not evenly balanced across the country. It probably never will be. There are pockets of overservice and underservice almost everywhere. Recent figures have shown that the United States has one physician for every 500 people; the figures also showed, however, that Washington, D.C. has one for every 175 people, whereas South Dakota has one for every 950. Even within a single city the supply/demand equation can change dramatically from one part of town to another. Underservice may be severe in an inner city ghetto, whereas the wealthy suburbs are inundated with physicians. Moreover, the demand in a particular area for physicians in general may belie the need for a particular specialty.

These facts tell you very little, however. Knowing about raw need tells you little about attitude or area dynamics; needless to say, all three factors are important. It may seem irrational, but you may interview for a position in underserved rural areas where the local medical community tries to lock you out, or in physician-rich areas where a group is more than welcoming.

Despite the burgeoning oversupply of physicians, intelligent, assiduous exploration of opportunities in areas of particular interest will likely turn up a reasonably lucrative and satisfying position. Keep in mind that you need only one job, so the gross numbers that indicate an overloaded profession mean little. With patience and a little luck, you can take advantage of the old saw, "Statistics don't apply to the individual."

Specialty Imbalance

Medicine is no longer a single discipline (if it ever was); it is a collection of distinct specialties, and different specialists require different numbers of patients for adequate support. In practical terms, this statement is illustrated by the fact that an area of 50,000 people may have one neurosurgeon and ten internists—and be underserved in terms of internists. The demographic, economic, and cultural characteristics of a community impact powerfully on the demand for medical services. An upper middle class community, for instance, supports more dermatologists than a lower middleclass area, regardless of what the standard physician/patient ratios for dermatologists lead you to expect.

Geographic imbalances exist across specialties and may be pronounced in a given state, county, or community. To assess the need for your skills in an area you prefer, you must examine the physician/patient ratios for your specialty and for specialties on which you might depend for referrals, not just ratios for physicians in general. If there are numerous physicians but few radiologists and radiology is your field, the surfeit of other physicians is actually to your advantage.

Too Many Physicians?

If you are despairing over the diminished demand for physician services, keep in mind that such demand can flow as rapidly as it can ebb. The inexorable aging of the baby boomers, the public demand for stricter regulation of physicians, and increasing restrictions on foreign medical graduates are forces that can substantially boost demand or lower supply.

Moreover, the development of new technologies is broadening the capabilities of and demand for certain specialties—witness what the evolution of new imaging modalities did for radiologists—and will undoubtedly create new demands and whole new specialties.

In other words, even though you are entering the job market at an inopportune time, you can find a suitable place almost without question. Furthermore, it is a waste of time and energy to worry about the future. It is impossible to predict it, and you certainly have little influence on the major forces likely to affect it.

Market Area Profile

In 1985 the American Medical Association (AMA) launched a program called the Market Area Profile (MAP). As the name indicates, a MAP supplies demographics on areas nationwide—anywhere you might consider settling into a practice. For example, a MAP for a ten-mile radius of a certain town reports the population there, the number of households, and the number of those households that are families. It also states the number of physicians in that radius and categorizes them by specialty and age.

The MAP includes the population, projections of population growth, and doctor/patient ratios for each specialty. It characterizes the people in the area by age group. For example, perhaps the average resident in the area of interest is 35 years old: 28% are younger than 21; 19% are 65+; and 34% of the women are between 21 and 44. MAP also provides trends—projected figures for four years.

The profile looks at the local hospitals: the number of admissions last year, the number of births, and a breakdown by specialty of doctors with admitting privileges. It lists specialties but not subspecialties. It gives the number of dermatologists in an area, for example, but not the number who specialize in dermatologic surgery. It does not list the business hours of competing physicians, or the facilities of the various offices, e.g. laboratories or radiographic capabilities. It does, however, include information about the existence of free-standing ambulatory centers and health maintenance organizations (HMOs) in the area.

The economics of an area are also included in the profile. It gives the unemployment rate for men of working age, the median household income, the number of households with incomes below $10,000, and the number of persons on Medicaid.

Despite the valuable information derived from a MAP, it does not replace basic legwork. It makes no projections (apart from population trends) about future needs or demand for medical care in the area and tells you nothing about the subspecialty interests and activities of established practitioners. For example, one of the general internists in a community may have developed a special interest in cardiology. He has attended many meetings and has made a major investment in noninvasive diagnostic equipment. You, as a fellowship-trained noninvasive cardiologist moving into the community, would face stiff resistance from such an individual. This situation cannot be anticipated from the MAP data or any other area statistics.

Other Assessment Maneuvers

When it comes to assessing a community of particular interest to you, keep in mind that large-area statistics may misrepresent the picture in a particular locale. Nothing substitutes for intelligent, on-site legwork. In a small area, for example, the attitude and subspecialty interests of established practitioners or the addition or loss of one or two physicians can dramatically affect the need for your services.

Even if you settle in an area overdoctored in your specialty, it is possible to do well if you choose the proper location. For instance, a moderate-sized, rapidly growing city may have a glut of physicians, but not one of them has located his office in the path of recent suburban expansion. If you are the first to do so, chances are you will be busy quickly, while your downtown colleagues stumble over themselves in search of patients.

Never underestimate the power of *intangibles* such as personality, political savvy, shared background and interests, and contacts from medical school or postgraduate training programs for attracting referrals from local colleagues. The presence or absence of these factors, which can make or break you in a community, can be evaluated only by direct, on-site investigation.

Diversification of Practices

Your job-hunting spirit should be buoyed by the ever-widening range of professional opportunities available in today's marketplace. The diversity is far greater today than even ten years ago. HMO positions, for example, were available only in selected areas a decade ago; today they are available in virtually every large community. Emergency room positions have also become commonplace over the same span of time, while urgent-care centers and locum tenens opportunities have added to the diversity of clinical jobs. Even more recently, newly created positions in medical management represent an evolving discipline for physicians and an expanding segment of the job market.

Certain types of positions evolve and change character over time. As a case in point, academic job roles have changed considerably as the ebb of federal funds for research has forced changes in the mix of research, teaching, and clinical work required of academicians.

The expansion in both the range and the diversity of professional opportunities has the disadvantage of creating confusion in the minds of the typical job hunter. On the other hand, it has the advantage of increasing the probability that the conscientious physician can more accurately match his needs and aspirations with the characteristics of a particular practice. The extent to which the bewildering array of options either comforts or confounds you depends on the care and conscientiousness you bring to the task of understanding the possibilities.

Trend Toward Group Practice

By the mid-1990s, most physicians across the United States will practice in groups, rather than solo or in pairs. One-third of them already do, and in certain areas the proportion is well beyond one-half. The fact that a much higher percentage of younger physicians practice in groups compared with their older colleagues adds confidence to the prediction that the current trend toward groups as the preferred mode of medical practice is likely to continue.

This trend is as recent as it is dramatic. At the end of World War II there were fewer than a dozen groups in the United States with more than 25 physicians. A group of 15 physicians would have been considered "large." Today "large" means at least 40 to 50 physicians; and if the trend toward increasing size continues, it may soon refer only to groups with more than 100 members.

The pace of expansion in both the number and size of medical groups picked up during the early 1980s. In 1984, according to the American Medical Association, there were well over 15,000 groups (defined as three or more doctors, formally organized), up from fewer than 11,000 in 1980—a jump of 44%. Over the same period, the number of group positions ballooned from 88,000 to 140,000, with the average size of each practice increasing from 8.2 to 9.1 physicians. This figure probably exceeds 10.0 today.

Single-specialty groups dominate the group practice landscape, representing more than 70% of all groups, up from 50% in 1969. The increase in the size of medical groups, however, has been especially pronounced in multispecialty practices, where the average number of positions jumped from 10 in 1969 to 27 in 1984. (*Future Practice Alternatives in Medicine*, Nash, D.B. ed, IGAKU-SHOIN, New York, pp. 16–17)

There are several factors behind these trends, including patients, hospitals, third party payers, the growing cost and complexity of operating a business, and the burgeoning debt of medical school graduates—not to mention the preferences of the physicians themselves.

Patients are more savvy about the medical marketplace than ever before and recognize that a large clinic generally has a better ability to provide comprehensive care, which also precludes their having to go to numerous places for tests, procedures, and consultations. Megaclinics tend to build reputations that attract patients and perpetuate themselves.

It has been estimated that the nation's 5000 hospitals amount to 2500 too many. Therefore *hospitals*, in the scramble to save their own lives, are "joint-venturing" in every conceivable direction. The idea is to fill their beds, use their resources, and make themselves essential to the community. The question is with whom are they to joint-venture? The answer is large group practices. The groups have the physicians and the business acumen. The group member who proposes a viable business idea to a hospital is likely to find himself president of the enterprise—backed by hospital money. Moreover, new ventures attract new physicians and new patients, satisfying all concerned.

The trend toward *third party payers* contracting with groups to care for their enrollees is also fueling the trend toward more and larger groups. Medicare and other large payers already have several hundred thousand beneficiaries enrolled in HMOs, preferred provider organizations (PPOs), independent practice associations (IPAs), and the like; many states are steering their burdensome Medicaid plans that way as well. As power in the medical industry shifts from provider to consumer, groups must adapt themselves to payer demands, and physicians must go where the patients are.

The factors just outlined draw many young *physicians* to the group setting, but others find that the cost and complexity of establishing a solo practice today seals their decision. When setting up a practice, the array of issues alone can be daunting, especially considering how ill-prepared we are to address them: As a new practitioner you must hire, train, and supervise personnel; price your services and collect your fees; choose a location; build or rent space; and buy or lease furniture and equipment, including telephones, typewriters, computers, diagnostic equipment, medical records, billing forms, file cabinets, floor covering, desks, examination tables, chairs, stationary, plants, and pictures—everything necessary to outfit your waiting room, examination rooms, laboratory, business office, reception area, and of course your private office. It is enough to stymie all but the most committed.

If you manage to get past the complexity issue, you are likely to become impaled on the cost. The typical physician emerges from residency $40,000 to $60,000 in debt, making the cost of setting up and equipping a new solo practice—usually $50,000 to $150,000 or more—prohibitive without at least some financial support from a sponsor. The risk is heightened by the sobering fact that success in practice is less certain now than ever before.

The influx of women to the profession is another factor. Women physicians are more likely than their male counterparts to work as employees, to join groups; recruiters say also that women are willing to accept smaller salaries. In return, groups are increasingly willing to make scheduling concessions to accommodate women with families. The availability of locum tenens coverage even makes it feasible for groups to offer meaningful amounts of maternity leave.

Also influencing the growth of group practice is the fact that the younger generation of physicians does not have the single-minded professional focus or the rugged-individualist mentality their fathers brought to the profession. Not surprisingly, physicians under age 40 are more likely than their older colleagues to associate with medical groups.

Young physicians not only tend to practice more sophisticated and defensive medicine, they face a bigger menu of life choices. They must deal with changing roles and relationships at home, at work, and in the community, which places great demands on their time and energy.

Without making value judgments, it is probably fair to say that young physicians tend to view medicine as one of several important dimensions in their lives and less as a mission or calling. They view it more as a job—an excellent job to be sure—but something to walk away from at times, take vacation from, not to marry and live with every minute of every day. Thus young physicians in particular gravitate to groups not only for the traditional clinical reasons of collegial support, consultation, and referral but also for fewer hours, for more structured work and call schedules, and to free themselves from the time requirements associated with the business aspects of medical practice.

Practices from Which to Choose

The remainder of this chapter is devoted to highlighting some of the key advantages and disadvantages—the "tradeoffs," if you will—of various practice types. The discussion is hampered, however, by the absence of a meaningful taxonomy of medical practice. For example, distinguishing among solo, two-person, and group practice (as is traditional) seems far less useful than viewing medical practice on a continuum, from a one-person practice to the practice that encompasses more than 100 physicians. The advantages and disadvantages of each type of practice vary as a function of practice size and setting. Therefore the arbitrary distinction between "solo," "partnership," and "group" practice serves little purpose and may confuse more than contribute to the discussion.

For example, a three-person, fee-for-service, single-specialty "group" represents tradeoffs that are surely closer to those found in solo practice than those found in a huge, prepaid, multispecialty "group." A group of surgeons based in a private, suburban hospital faces a different set of advantages and disadvantages than a similar size group of radiologists practicing in a free-standing surgicenter or a university teaching institution.

In other words, the context, or "environment," of the practice and how the practice relates to its environment can have as much influence on the group as any intrinsic factor. This point is especially true for the issue of how the group relates to the "market" for its services. Does the group prefer to operate in the "open" market with fee-for-service payments from an undefined patient population, or does it care for a defined patient population that it serves on a prepaid, capitated basis according to some "managed care" arrangement?

The following overview is meant to be used in conjunction with the self-knowledge you gained from the previous chapter. Taken together, the insights from the two chapters should help you position yourself in the most appropriate category of professional opportunities. Once you decide (with the help of Chapter 5) on the type or category of practice likely to suit you best, you are ready to choose a specific opportunity from the many you deem generally appropriate and suitable to who you are and what you want out of life (see Chapter 3). At that point, the tools available to you in Chapters 6, 7, and 8 will help you find and evaluate specific opportunities and then negotiate a favorable arrangement with the practice you prefer.

SOLO PRACTICE

The solo physician is traditionally a rugged individualist. Although solo practice has receded in importance, it has long been the predominant means of delivering care. Despite the growing importance of group practice, nearly 40% of nonfederally employed physicians (excluding residents) in patient care still practice solo. (*Physician Employment Patterns: Challenging Conventional Wisdom* by W. D. Marder, *Health Affairs*, People to People Health Foundation, Inc., Millwood, Va., Winter 1988)

The percent of physicians practicing alone varies widely by specialty. More than 50% of surgeons and self-employed psychiatrists practice solo, but fewer than 9% of radiologists and pathologists choose that form of practice. General internists and family practitioners, who together make up the bulk of clinicians, practice solo 41% and 45% of the time, respectively. (*Physician Employment Patterns: Challenging Conventional Wisdom* by W. D. Marder, *Health Affairs*, People to People Health Foundation, Inc., Millwood, Va., Winter 1988).

Solo practice is for the person with a strong ego and work ethic, a desire for high income, and a need for maximum autonomy and independence; he likes calling the shots and not having to reconcile his needs and wants with those of anyone else. He is a self-starter who can keep himself motivated and on track, even through adversity, without collegial feedback and support.

In return for the independence and autonomy, however, he foregoes the quick consults in difficult situations and the sympathetic ear on difficult days. He not uncommonly gives up his personal life and marries his job. In that sense his independence may be more apparent than real, as his practice is a major commitment and often a confinement. The time demands on a solo practitioner can be consuming.

He is vulnerable to a variety of patient demands, including phone calls at any hour, even if it is just from the emergency room physician to report about a patient. A group of doctors might hire a nurse specifically to field calls and dispense advice throughout the day, but the solo practitioner probably cannot afford it, at least not at first, and likely would not have the volume of incoming calls to justify it anyway. Therefore he fields the calls himself. At 6 p.m. of the typical day, he finds 15 messages on his desk and is tied there until 7:30 p.m. returning them. He may work out a call-sharing arrangement with colleagues, but because other physicians are basically his competitors, he may prefer to handle his on-call responsibilities himself.

A solo physician had better be a good business manager, too, because a practice is a business and must be managed as one, at least if it is to achieve a reasonable measure of financial success. Here, too, a physician may not have the financial resources for support or consultation beyond the basics of having someone help set up the books.

In short, he has to worry about everything himself. In today's practice, "everything" includes insurance procedures, billing and collecting, compliance with countless state and federal regulations, work flow, general office efficiency, payroll, hiring and firing, scheduling patients, the coffee machine, the cleaning crew, and building management. If he is less than effective in any facet, the deficiency shows up in that other major worry, the bottom line.

Thus solo practice is a tradeoff involving extremes. The income potential is open-ended, but so is the time demand. The solo practitioner is captain of his ship, but he must deal directly with the realities of being the boss. He is the sole beneficiary of the fruits of his labor, and solely liable for the entire business.

If that situation is for you, the next step is to take over or buy an existing practice, or you can start one from scratch. A practice broker can help you find one for sale. In certain, mostly smaller locations, local sponsors (e.g. a community hospital or a regional committee formed to attract doctors) may provide financial backing.

Unless you secure financial guarantees from the community, you are at great financial risk when starting your own venture. Your investment comes at the front end (your start-up costs), but the *cash* does not start coming in until later. Cash flow is the lifeblood of any business; therefore you had better have adequate financing to bridge the gap. It also behooves you to be especially careful when assessing the local supply of and demand for your specialty, and the attitude of established physicians about your joining their community; a practice in its formative period is particularly sensitive to these forces.

Current trends in medical practice seem destined to make solo practitioners a vanishing breed, perhaps to be found principally among older physicians and in rural communities. Nevertheless, these trends can be changed by forces not now evident. Nothing remains static.

GROUP PRACTICE

"Group practice" covers an enormous range of professional situations, from three doctors to more than 100; from single-specialty groups to some that cover every discipline in medicine; from the fee-for-service payment method to capitated, prepaid care to mixtures of each in varying proportions; from institution-based groups of medical faculty personnel to community-based groups of physicians whose last involvement with an academic institution was the day they left residency.

It is not surprising that no one has developed a good taxonomy of practice types. In the face of such diversity, it is difficult to identify characteristics associated with group practice in general. Nonetheless, there are some general statements that can give you a sense of what to expect.

Broadly, group practice is characterized by the notion of sharing. You and your colleagues share risks, costs, responsibilities, and rewards. The notion implies a communal situation that must be understood and respected. You receive collegial support, have structured hours, and are responsible for only limited call, but you cannot hire and fire whom you please, and you must practice your specialty according to agreed-upon norms of what is reasonable and acceptable, not your own notions. You gain support but lose autonomy. That is the essence of group practice.

Often associated with group practice is the notion of limitation of risk. There is certainly less financial risk and often no risk in terms of purchasing a building, furniture, or equipment. Data on physician earnings suggest that doctors in fee-for-service group practices have larger incomes than solo practitioners, probably owing in large measure to the greater revenue generated by ancillary services in group practices. More than 50% of groups have electrocardiography capabilities, radiology services, and clinical laboratories, many of which are elaborate; so, not surprisingly, average revenue per patient contact is higher in group practice than in a solo or a two-person practice.

A final noteworthy and generally applicable characteristic of group practice is the idea of peer review, a shared standard of acceptable medical performance. Although the solo physician is not entirely free of peer scrutiny, such scrutiny does not occur as directly or extensively as it generally does when you practice in a group, elbow to elbow with other doctors. Depending on your perspective, peer review can be somewhat threatening, or it can be a source of comfort, reassurance, and security.

In this era of having to define and adhere to "community standards" of care to avoid malpractice litigation and losses, peer review is especially helpful. It is readily available in the group practice situation and therefore more apt to be used. Colleagues can quickly and informally confirm or deny each other's diagnostic thinking or treatment strategy. Physicians in a large group often become increasingly specialized and, ideally, their expertise is shared with their colleagues.

As a general rule, the larger the group, the greater the potential for realizing these advantages. With increased group size, however, comes increased complexity and diffusion of authority and responsibility. The larger the group, the more you must subordinate your needs and preferences to group rules and routines.

In the largest, most bureaucratic groups, the physician is just a midlevel cog in the wheel, much like the anonymous lawyer in a large law firm. Regardless of your status—partner or hourly worker—your role is defined like any other employee's role. You conform to the group's standard procedures, or you leave. In the not-too-distant future, you may even find yourself practicing according to clinical protocols and to increasingly rigid criteria for resource utilization.

Typically, the larger the group, the larger the role and power of those involved in the management and business end of the practice.

Management could be by committee or by dictatorship. The managers could be medical colleagues or business types with MBAs (masters degrees in business administration). The practice might be driven by professional values or by business imperatives. In an excellent discussion in the *Milbank Quarterly* (Donald L. Madison and Thomas R. Konrad, Cambridge University Press, New York, NY, 1988) Madison and Konrad used the apt term "organizational culture" to describe these issues and emphasized their importance for understanding the relationship between the physician and the organization to which he belongs.

Central to the issue of organizational culture is the organization's beliefs about the proper rank, status, prerogatives, and obligations of its physicians. Madison and Konrad emphasized that these beliefs differ markedly from one organization to the next, and they recommended using professional autonomy—at the level of both the individual physician and the medical staff as a whole—as one of two key dimensions for characterizing medical groups. The other dimension is the extent to which a group's service capacity is "committed" (already spoken for) under any kind of consumer affiliation arrangement or prepayment contract. Student Health Services, a government care program, and "closed panel" HMOs represent extreme examples wherein the organization's entire service capacity is committed in advance.

The key question is the extent to which the medical staff or its representatives determine the values, priorities, and initiatives—the goals—of the organization. Do doctors run the show and control their own destiny, or are they beholden to some higher authority, such as a group of investors, government officials, representatives of a religious order, or a hospital board?

In short, then, the relationship between a group and its physicians, revolving around the issue of professional autonomy and power, is central to the group's organizational culture, which in turn is a key determinant of the tradeoffs that accrue to physicians with membership in the group.

HOSPITAL-BASED PRACTICE

The hospital-based practice often but not always involves an employment relationship between hospital and physician, the physician usually being a radiologist, anesthesiologist, pathologist, or emergency room specialist. Even if the physician practices as an independent contractor on a fee-for-service basis, the hospital may be involved in his billing and collections. The relationship functions, in effect, as an employment relationship but with the physician retaining certain professional prerogatives.

A distinguishing characteristic of this form of practice is that the workplace, some or all of the equipment, and many or all of the employees with whom you work are provided or leased to you by the hospital—hence the great potential for conflict between organizational and professional interests.

For example, the radiologists of a hospital may be members of an independent group practice, but the technologists on whom they depend are employed by the hospital. Who controls the technologists' work—the physicians or the hospital administrator? Because the physicians are responsible for the quality of care they provide, they must have a certain degree if not complete control over the technologists. The problem lies with the fact that the technologists work for, are paid by, and therefore are subject to control by the administrator.

In some instances the potential conflict is circumvented by an agreement giving the physician the right to have an employee discharged when, in his judgment, quality of care is at stake. With the example given, it is easy to understand why, when considering a hospital-based practice, it is important to understand how these issues are handled in that particular setting.

In another situation, the radiologists may complain that an aging piece of equipment is no longer state-of-the-art, and the administrator might argue that the budget does not allow a new one. He might ask, "What would it contribute to the bottom line—the income of my institution?" A Pinto, after all, gets you from one place to another as well as a Benz.

In the emergency room, the administrator may urge the nursing staff to "accommodate" as many patients per hour as possible. Speed, efficiency, and revenue are important business goals for him and the hospital, so he leans on the staff—his employees—to maximize them. By contrast, the emergency room physicians may be working on fixed incomes from the group that provides the hospital's emergency coverage, and thus have little motivation to see more patients per hour. Income aside, they are primarily concerned with quality of care, which is seldom the ally of speed.

In the anesthesiology field, controversy currently rages over (1) the number of certified registered nurse anesthetists (CRNAs) an anesthesiologist can effectively supervise; (2) if the anesthesiologist can supervise and administer anesthesia concurrently; and for that matter (3) if CRNAs need any physician supervision at all. The administrator of a hospital that cannot attract enough anesthesiologists to handle the volume of surgery performed may want to hire CRNAs to keep the operating rooms busy. Anesthesiologists, on the other hand, may believe that CRNAs should not practice without proper supervision. (In most venues the anesthesiologist is legally responsible for the CRNAs' work.) Therefore the anesthesiologist may be unwilling to administer and supervise concurrently, and wants to limit the number of CRNAs to whatever number he can properly supervise—which may comprise fewer than those needed to keep the surgical suites humming.

In areas where CRNAs can practice independently, turf battles between physician anesthesiologists and CRNAs can be fierce. Too many naive physicians, believing that training and expertise would prevail over "petty politics," have been run out of town by an entrenched group of CRNAs whose power they underestimated.

Another potentially major conflict throughout the profession that is even more acute in hospital-based practice comes from reimbursement schemes based on diagnostic-related groups (DRGs). Before DRGs, hospitals and doctors espoused the same goal: the best possible care at *any* cost. Indeed they shared the financial incentive to approach health care with that attitude. Hospitals were paid on a cost-plus reimbursement basis; so the more costs their physicians generated, the more income they received. Fee-for-service physicians were reimbursed almost open-endedly for whatever charges they generated. Therefore the more services the better—certainly for the physicians, the hospital, and presumably the patient, but not for the payers (employers, insurers, and Uncle Sam).

In part through the DRGs, payers have begun to assert themselves. Hospitals are no longer paid cost-plus for Medicare patients but receive instead a fixed stipend for each case, based on the DRG within which it falls. Profit no longer comes from increasing the charges but from treating the patient and closing out the case before costs outrun the stipend or budget. DRGs have forced hospitals to look at the practice style of their staff physicians with new eyes. Yesterday's hero—the physician who ran up charges—is today's villain, as the more tests and procedures he generates the more he stresses the DRG budgets and the more profit he saps from the hospital.

The DRGs have forced hospitals to work in a more businesslike fashion by establishing budgets within which they must deliver services. Efficiency is the new key to remaining financially viable, and in the name of efficiency, hospital management is often forced to make difficult and sometimes unsavory tradeoffs between the quality and the cost of care.

The remark that physicians are being encouraged to discharge patients "quicker and sicker" is an outgrowth of the DRG-inspired pressure to release patients a day or two sooner than doctors might deem optimal in order to save the cost of two inpatient days. Since DRGs have appeared on the scene, hospital administrators seem to believe that patients "prefer to recover at home."

There is yet another potential conflict connected with hospital-based practice in the era of DRGs. Let us say that a fee-for-service radiologist group wants a new $2 million magnetic resonance scanner, explaining to the administrator how superior the images are to those obtainable with the old computed tomography machine. Although they do not emphasize the point, the radiologists may also be thinking of the additional fees the new equipment would generate for them. In the past, the administrator probably would have liked the idea, as the expenditure would have increased the hospital's reimbursements from third-party payers. Today, the money would most likely come from the hospital's capital budget, which probably is funded from revenues or from debt financing. The administrator now views the new machine as just more overhead, not a reimbursable cost, and therefore tells the radiologists that the hospital cannot afford it.

Yet another situation, which can be described as diabolical, occurs when the hospital pressures a physician, however subtly, to change his characterization of a patient's illness and call it something that garners a larger DRG stipend. Changing a patient's "primary" diagnosis, often a matter of some conjecture, can substantially affect DRG payments. There are even computer programs available that can maximize DRG revenue by "optimizing" the rank order of established medical diagnoses. This situation is an important one to ponder because when the physician is not wholly independent of the hospital, the potential exists for undue influence by the hospital on his professional judgment and decisions.

INSTITUTIONAL POSITIONS

By accepting institutional employment, you are moving into an organizational environment where the delivery of medical services is but a small part of the organization's activity.

Company Physician

The occupational physician customarily provides "urgent," or walk-in type care for company personnel. He has an office on or near the company grounds, and he practices with an eye toward minimizing job hazards and occupational risk to the employees.

The potential for conflict between the needs and rights of the employer and those of the sick employee is obvious. The challenge to the company physician is one of finding common ground between the goals of the two parties, or when that is not possible, striving for sensible, reasonable tradeoffs between disparate goals. The appropriately trained physician is in a particularly good position to meet such a challenge.

At best, the practice of occupational medicine is based on a solid commitment to preventive medicine. Occupational physicians have an excellent opportunity to work with a relatively healthy, alert, productive patient population and to contribute to the health and welfare of a potentially large number of patients by thoughtful, effective policy formulation.

The company physician, however, is not the patient's primary physician, so most medical problems, with the exception of hypertension and drug abuse, are diagnosed and treated by outside physicians. Opportunities for hands-on diagnosis and treatment are therefore severely limited.

The company physician is a salaried employee whose income and benefits are well defined by the company's wage and salary guidelines. There is no overhead, no insurance worry, and little in the way of production pressure. In all likelihood, a company physician has the luxury of taking as much time as he would like to counsel patients. He also has structured, limited hours and virtually no on-call responsibilities.

CLINICAL INVESTIGATOR

Usually employed by pharmaceutical firms, the clinical investigator is involved in research and administration, with little or no patient care. He sets up and oversees clinical trials involving well defined protocols for animal or human testing of new drugs. A peculiar characteristic of these positions is that travel can be extensive, as much of the selling and supervision of these often large-scale clinical trials take place in academic institutions and private offices around the United States.

As with company physicians, clinical investigators are salaried employees whose income and benefit package is defined by institutional wage and salary guidelines. They are also free of financial risks, billing and collection hassles, and malpractice worries.

ACADEMIC PHYSICIAN

Academic positions have high social value and prestige. Under the right circumstances, they can provide exciting professional stimulation, including teaching opportunities and a chance to contribute to society in ways beyond the one-on-one doctor-patient interaction. In the heyday of federal funding for medical schools, academic positions could be geared largely or entirely to research and teaching. Federal funding declined during the 1980s, however, and academic positions have increasingly come to resemble positions in the private sector but with much lower pay. Time for research and teaching has been curtailed as faculty members are pressured to generate more and more of their compensation from clinical revenue.

Promotion and tenure within the institution, however, are still based on the system of "publish or perish." For the academician of the 1980s and 1990s, clinical time and teaching cut into time for research and writing, but research and writing remain essential to career advancement. With demands and incentives often in conflict, academic positions can play havoc with your equilibrium. Moreover, you may spend intolerable amounts of time sitting in committee meetings which, as with most bureaucracies, are likely to be long and tiresome.

Despite its disadvantages, academic positions still offer rewards available nowhere else in the profession, including the opportunity to contribute to society in the broadest possible way by developing new knowledge and by shaping the clinical skills of young physicians.

GOVERNMENT AND MILITARY PRACTICE

Military positions represent all the advantages and disadvantages of operating within the largest, most bureaucratic of environments. Military medical practice is directed by policies and procedures that reduce uncertainties and establish priorities and predictability. The size and rigidly hierarchical structure of such organizations severely limit your flexibility and input about how things are done. In the military, minimal autonomy also means that you have little or no say over where you can live and work: You go where you are ordered to go.

In return, however, you have the security offered by the organization. Although you cannot aspire to high income, you never have to compete in the marketplace or worry about the company going broke. Furthermore, pensions are generous. Today, the greatest advantage of government practice may be that it is the one safe harbor from malpractice for physicians in clinical practice.

Basically, the military represents the ultimate tradeoff between autonomy and security. Depending on your personality, it could represent a good tradeoff, or it could be a nightmare.

Unfortunately, there is one more thing you give up—a measure of professional respect from your peers. Many physicians view military medicine with a healthy dose of skepticism. Even if you practice the finest medicine anywhere, as is surely possible in military and Veterans Administration hospitals, you must contend with colleagues who believe that military medicine is to medicine as military music is to music.

LOCUM TENENS

At the opposite extreme from military practice is locum tenens, a form of medical practice virtually unknown in the United States a decade ago. It offers advantages virtually unavailable anywhere else in the profession.

Although you can certainly do locum tenens on your own, most physicians engaged in this form of practice work with organized, nationwide services, the best of which function like "geographically dispersed" group practices. These organizations match the skills and interest of their locum tenens staff with the needs of their clients. They arrange travel, housing, licensure, and staff privileges for their physicians, and they provide malpractice insurance.

Key advantages of this form of practice include the freedom and flexibility to work as much or as little as you want, and the opportunity to broaden your professional experience by working in many different practices and communities. Thus locum tenens is favored by physicians just completing their training, who use locum tenens to explore a wide variety of places and practices or to learn more about opportunities of particular interest; physicians seeking a less rigorous professional schedule, generally to pursue nonmedical interests (travel, hobbies, avocations); and physicians in transition between jobs.

Matching What You Want With What Is Available

Having gotten this far in the book, you should have a pretty fair idea about the shape of your peg (you) and the hole (practice) it should fit into. Although we use this analogy, choosing the right practice is not as straightforward as "fitting a round peg in a round hole." The problem is that the shape of the peg and the hole rarely match perfectly. How then do you go about getting the best possible fit?

The first and perhaps most important step in searching for the "perfect" practice is realizing that it does not exist. Do not waste your time, like Didi and Gogo, waiting for Godot. Rather, realize that any practice opportunity requires you to make trade-offs and often requires some compromise between the ideal and the real. What you are seeking is the most favorable tradeoffs and the best compromises.

There is one area, however, where you cannot afford much compromise, and that is in finding a practice that fits well with your personality—who you are and how you like to function. This subject was discussed in Chapter 3 as level I, or "intrinsic" considerations. On this level—the level of your basic personality—the fit must be as close as possible. Fortunately, there are any number of opportunities that may resonate reasonably well with your personality and therefore allow you to function comfortably.

By understanding yourself and the advantages and disadvantages of the various practice types, you can begin to focus on certain opportunities and exclude others. At that point, you can concentrate on the type of community you would like to live in and search for suitable options in your preferred locations.

The final steps of choosing a practice are (1) evaluating each of your leading options in depth, (2) deciding on the tradeoffs and compromises you are willing to make, and (3) negotiating the best deal. At some point you must decide, all things considered, which of your leading options is best. Such a decision is rarely easy. Decide you must, however, so here are some guidelines on how to make a good decision.

Fact Versus Opinion

As Peter Drucker pointed out in his classic work *The Effective Executive* (Harper & Row, New York, 1967, pp. 113-165), most people who write about decision-making seem to believe that good decisions start with the relevant facts. That is all well and good if the facts are clear; usually they are not, at least not as clear as people's opinions about what the relevant facts are.

Often in medicine and even more commonly in business, the facts do not influence decision-making nearly as much as opinions or interpretations of what are regarded as the key facts. Moreover, most of us are capable of developing a factual basis of support for a position or opinion we already hold.

"Facts" can thus be more misleading than opinions because opinions are generally recognized for what they are, i.e., hypotheses that need to be tested against reality and confirmed, denied, or modified. Applied to the process of choosing a practice, this reasoning suggests that opinions provide a fairly good starting point for understanding the characteristics of the places and practices you are considering.

In other words, to understand the advantages and disadvantages of the practices you are contemplating, you must go beyond the glittering generalities gleaned from your reading on the subject and speak in depth with colleagues who have practice experience and, hopefully, well formulated opinions about what they have experienced. At best, your reading on the subject can provide you with an intelligent set of questions and a framework for processing the input from colleagues.

Of course, your own experience is the best way to gather information and gain insight into the practices you are considering. Experience allows you to form your own opinions and evaluate more intelligently the opinions of others.

Another benefit of talking at length with experienced colleagues or gaining your own experience in practices of particular interest is that you come to appreciate subtle issues that you might otherwise have overlooked. It is especially true if you work in different practices for short periods, several weeks or months, doing locum tenens with no commitment. A series of such experiences should make the advantages and disadvantages of each practice stand out in bold relief.

Talking with colleagues, especially about the particulars of a given situation, has the additional advantage of allowing you to distinguish between generic situations and exceptions, another important element of good decision-making. Because something is generally true does not mean that it is true in a specific practice. Always reconcile your expectations of what *should* hold true with people's opinion about what *is* true for the situation at hand, and verify the opinions of others with your own observations. For example, there are certain things you expect to hold true, in general, for all group practices, such as the expectation of collegial support and consultation. In certain groups, though, personality clashes and political infighting may have long ago destroyed any semblance of support or cooperation among its members.

Opinions in decision-making are like hypotheses in science: They must be tested against reality. The question remains "whose reality?" In this case, the proving ground is your own experience. After all, it is your life. The richer and broader your "real world" experience, the better prepared you are to evaluate the input of others and make your own decision about which practice is right for you.

Soliciting opinions contributes to good decision-making in yet another way: It evokes disagreement and debate. When you speak with people, encourage them to offer clear opinions and challenge them to react to the opinions of others. Discussion and debate lead to better decisions by bringing different points of view into sharper focus and allowing you to choose the one you believe is best after carefully considering the range of opinions.

Finally, keep in mind that no matter how conscientious you are in gathering opinions, the end result is still a rather small data set—and we all know how unreliable small-sample research can be. Despite a few caveats concerning the opinions of experienced colleagues, getting others' opinions is nevertheless crucial to making a good decision. It is a good starting point.

Long-Term Versus Short-Term Perspective

A good decision is one based on a balance of factors. For example, immediate needs should be weighed against long-term desires. Considering the rate at which almost everything changes, you should probably "discount" future considerations. That is, the further into the future you project, the more uncertain your projection and therefore the less likely you are to feel the same way, have the same values, and want the same things when you reach that point in time.

Do not view any decision as immutable. You have years of professional life ahead, and you will witness many changes in that time. The structure of the medical marketplace is constantly changing, and your medical skills and interests are certain to evolve. There will also be changes in your desire for professional stimulation, your need for income, your recreational and social patterns, and your family structure.

In short, the practice you choose need not be forever, so do not act as if it were. Most physicians make at least one or two significant professional moves during their careers. Ideally, your moves will be changes for the better, initiated by you, not ones imposed by others or suffered as a result of bad decisions.

Therefore your soundest decisions are probably not ones based solely on a twenty-year perspective because you cannot possibly see clearly that far into the future. Nor should they be based solely on your immediate interests and preferences because they are likely to change. It is a question of balance.

One approach to the difficult task of balancing present and future considerations is the "don't burn your bridges" strategy. In essence, it suggests that you do what seems ideal now, or as far into the future as you are confident about, so long as it does not preclude options you might like to keep open further into the future. A corporate executive, for example, can always decide in midcareer to drop what he is doing and become a fishing guide, but a fishing guide cannot readily move from the streams and rivers into the executive suite. A professor of pediatrics can switch to solo practice on an Indian reservation, but a physician who spends the first 15 years of his career on a remote reservation cannot move directly from there to the post of department chairman.

Of course, you can easily carry that thinking too far, especially if you are accustomed, as most of us are, to postponing gratification. Learning to enjoy yourself today is as important as preparing for your future. At all points in your life, balance is as important as achievement if you want to keep your life on a reasonably even keel.

Trade-offs and Compromises

Accepting that there is no such thing as the perfect practice and that any decision must involve trade-offs and compromises, you should know how to make sensible trade-offs and good compromises. The notion of "compromise" is different from that "trade-off."

A *compromise* is a concession or adjustment, a thing intermediate between two things (e.g., a compromise solution) or a blending of the qualities of different things. When you compromise on something, the implication is that you did not get what you wanted; you settled for less. That is why compromises can be reasonable or poor, depending on the extent to which you had to sacrifice what you really wanted.

A *trade-off*, on the other hand, involves alternatives. No practice can possibly give you everything you want. One practice or location provides certain advantages and a different practice or location provides others. They are different, not better or worse.

The notion of alternatives suggests substituting certain things of value for other things of equal value. In the best possible light, it is like the child in the candy shop who has a wealth of wonderful choices but, alas, cannot have them all: His bag holds only so much candy. Such a situation requires that you narrow the options and choose those that are most appealing or important.

You may or may not have to compromise when choosing a practice; probably you will, to a greater or lesser extent. You surely will have to make trade-offs, as with virtually everything in life. The question is *which* trade-offs will you choose to make. Such decisions must be based on your values and preferences. Probably the worst mistake you could make at this juncture is to try to anticipate and respond to someone else's notions of what you should do or what should be important to you. As Polonius told his son, "To thine own self be true."

Compromises, on the other hand, can be good or bad depending on the extent to which you sacrificed or settled for less than you wanted. To distinguish good from bad compromises, you must be clear about your objective: What are you trying to accomplish? What need, interest, or goal are you trying to satisfy?

If, for example, your objective is to feed yourself, and someone offers you half a loaf of bread rather than a whole one, you say "yes," as half a loaf is a reasonable compromise: It is food, and it nourishes. Recall now the story of Solomon, who was asked to decide which of two mothers claiming the same baby had the legitimate claim. Solomon asked both women, at a signal, to pull on either side of the child so each could try to wrest the child away. As the wise king anticipated, the real mother let go. Half a baby is no compromise at all—it is a corpse, not half of a living human being.

A good compromise is one that preserves, to the extent possible, your fundamental interests, the goal that underlies the position you have staked out. If your goal is to pay off your debts within your first year of practice or it is to buy a home, you have flexibility when negotiating compensation up to the point that you simply will not have sufficient income to realize your goal. The compromise might be to accept the idea of a smaller house than you had planned on.

It is well to think through beforehand where and to what extent you are willing to compromise and what you are willing to trade off. What if a prestigious faculty offers you tenure, but you must sacrifice either teaching, research, or clinical work?—you cannot do all three. Which is it going to be? Such decisions are more intelligently made if you have thought things through in advance.

You can facilitate the process of making trade-offs and crafting compromises by clarifying your goals and prioritizing your needs, wants, and preferences. *Prioritizing* is based on the obvious notion that not all needs, values, and preferences have equal weight. Only you can decide how they rank. Be true to yourself. It is crucial here that you listen to your own inclinations, not someone else's. Make a list of your priorities, or at least have the top few clearly in mind. Such formulations allow you to begin the process of winnowing out the obviously bad fits among your various practice options and puts you in some reasonable area wherein lie the options most likely to be gratifying and fulfilling. Once you have reached that stage, narrowing the options and finalizing the decision may require further compromises and trade-offs.

- How does the importance of family life compare to the importance you place on your work? If autonomy and money are both important to you and a given practice situation offered you both, would you be willing to work long hours, take frequent call, and give up time with your two young daughters?
- How compelling is your need for other people? Must you work with others, do you need their support, their feedback? How do those needs and desires stack up against your desire for freedom and your irritation at rules and regulations?
- Do you want more money or more free time? Autonomy or collegial involvement? Research or clinical work? Suturing lacerations and passing out cold remedies in a walk-in center or monitoring critically ill patients in the intensive care unit?
- Where do you want to live? The established, expensive Northeast corridor or the wild, wide open West? You want your children to grow up with the cultural amenities of the urban environment, but are you willing to have them exposed to crime, drugs, and smog? Must you stay close to your family, or would you take a great opportunity 1000 miles away and make do with occasional visits and numerous long distance calls?
- You may want to be highly visible in your community, but can you tolerate being interrupted in restaurants by patients stopping by to update you on their condition?
- You can get an endowed chair at another university, but the change

requires you to sacrifice half the time you had for research, the beautiful garden you spent years cultivating, and your spouse's outstanding job? Is is worth it?

These questions are only a few of those that could be addressed. Life is full of trade-offs and compromises. The emphasis here is that you cannot avoid them, you simply have to make them. The key to making them wisely lies in getting to know who you are, how you like to function, what you want and what you value—establishing priorities.

Healthy people accept that they cannot have it all. Therefore when choosing a practice, the question is to what extent you have to compromise what you want or value, or for that matter who you are and how you like to function. On key issues, you simply cannot compromise much and expect to be happy. You must find a situation that permits you to function comfortably, where your basic need for support, feedback, autonomy, freedom, structure, or whatever, can be satisfied.

Perhaps you are a leader, a doer, someone who likes to inspire others, take charge and make things happen, get things done. If you find a position in which you can function that way, chances are you will be fairly effective and happy, regardless of the context or the compromises you may have to make in other respects. You may be willing, for example, to put up with the extra hours, the paperwork, politics, and committee meetings expected of someone in your position, if it is a position you strived for and attained because it allowed you to express and experience yourself in ways that are important to you.

Perhaps you are highly ambitious. The question is then in what arena can your ambition blossom and lead you to satisfying and successful endeavors? If you are the outgoing, gregarious type, you might be stimulated by the politicking and speech-making required of a medical director or department chairman, the very requirements that would be highly stressful to the shy, retiring person.

If you are the shy, retiring type, you might direct your ambition toward something different, such as winning government grants or a Research Scientist Award, both which require hour upon hour of painstaking, solitary work in a laboratory or behind a desk. The combination of shyness and ambition fits better with being an ac-comlished researcher than a public figure.

The point is that your "intrinsic" needs and fundamental personal-ity are the most compelling considerations when determining how to position yourself in the real world. You cannot expect to go against the grain and be happy and comfortable. That is not to say that you cannot get away with it—just that you will pay a steep price.

By comparison, your "extrinsic" needs (see Chapter 3) can be traded off and compromised with relative abandon. If you do not make much money this year, there is always next year. If you were not able to send your children to private school, perhaps you can hire a tutor. If you miss the smell of salt air, perhaps the crisp, fresh smell of mountain meadows will substitute reasonably well. Living through another harsh winter is not the worst thing in the world— maybe you could take up skiing and learn to have fun in the snow.

Summary

When looking for the perfect practice, it is important to accept early on that it does not exist. Do not expect to find perfection. Do not doom yourself to waiting for something that is not coming down the road. Do not wait for Godot.

Concentrate on finding a practice that resonates with your person-ality type, that allows you to be who you are and to function com-fortably and effectively. You cannot afford to compromise much, if at all, on the level of your intrinsic needs or your basic values, prefer-ences, and personality.

After you decide what type or category of practice fits with who you are and what you really want out of life, you must develop opportunities within that universe of possibilities. Then, to narrow the options, you must decide what trade-offs and compromises you are willing to make. Trade-offs are a normal, expected part of choos-ing anything in life. For any path you pursue, there will always be "the road not taken." Prioritizing your extrinsic wants and desires should put you into a reasonably good position to evaluate your options and the trade-offs inherent in each.

Compromises are different in that a compromise requires that you accept less than what you wanted. Most choices in life involve some degree of compromise, your choice of where and how to practice included. By clarifying your short- and long-range goals, you can craft reasonable compromises that will preserve, to the extent possible, what is most important to you.

Trade-offs and compromises are inherent in all opportunities. The question is how much and what kind of each. By learning the art of negotiating, you can minimize the compromises and optimize the trade-offs. Before you can start negotiating, though, you must develop specific practice options and understand what each has to offer.

■ 6

Where to Look for a Job

Assuming that you do not intend to launch a solo practice or join your father, you will have to look for a position. Having learned the lessons of the previous chapters, you probably have at least a notion of the type or category of practice you want and the geographic/demographic area in which you wish to live. The question now is how to find a suitable position.

The immediate goal of your search is to maximize the number of opportunities that meet your requirements. Once that is done, you must evaluate each opportunity in some depth, separating the wheat from the chaff, to see which of the leading contenders makes an offer that suits you.

Developing Your Options

One method of searching is to use the *classifieds*. Although it is not the most efficient job-hunting strategy, investigating classified ads is far from worthless. Many good opportunities may be found there—if the opening is still available by the time you discover it.

A modern variant of classified advertising is direct mail advertising. This method became common during the 1980s, as computer typewriters and laser printers have made it cost-effective for all but the smallest companies, and even they can contract for direct mailing from firms that specialize in such services. Opportunities touted via direct mail may be "fresher," more apt to be available when you respond than ones depicted in the classifieds.

Do not expect to be able to distinguish good opportunities from bad from the ads themselves. If you use this method, be prepared for plenty of "legwork"—making the contacts, presenting yourself properly, evaluating the opportunities. These measures are essential if you want to maximize your chances of success.

Another way to explore job opportunities is to use a *medical-society placement service*. The utility of these services varies widely, generally in the fair to poor range, but nonetheless may be worth a try. "Placement service" is a misnomer. At best, they are matching services; at worst, they are out-of-date listings.

Certain specialty societies or colleges make available physician's names and perhaps abbreviated curricula vita to hiring authorities, and they provide a list of openings to job-seeking physicians. Such a service, however, has no real incentive to fill openings or place doctors.

A third job-hunting strategy is to use a *private placement service*. Compared with the passive job sources—classifieds, listings, postings, mail notices—a private placement service takes an active, interactional approach to finding you a position. An agency person goes about the task of finding and pursuing opportunities for you, sparing you much of the legwork. Agency personnel are fee-motivated professionals, and it is in their interest to place you. With rare exception, their fee is paid by the employer.

Many physicians believe that institutions or groups that must hire a search firm to fill their positions are lacking in some way. This attitude does not apply in today's world. In fact, search firms represent many outstanding institutions that simply do not have the time, inclination, or experience to recruit properly.

Networking is perhaps the most common way of finding a practice. Networking involves discovering opportunities and making yourself known to those in charge by word of mouth. To be maximally effective, this strategy requires a fairly well focused idea of the area, type of practice, and ideally even the specific group with which you would like to be associated.

The fifth and perhaps most "modern" strategy is to use *locum tenens*—a more proactive, self-directed variant of networking—to identify and pursue opportunities consistent with what you are looking for. Locum tenens has the advantage of allowing you to "audition" for openings in which you are interested. If you are uncertain about what you want, locum tenens can provide a taste of many places and practice situations, from which you can gain insight and information about the job market and your professional preferences.

The rest of the chapter takes a closer look at each of the basic five ways of exploring your options.

Classified Advertising

> Wanted: general internist, for three person group, lakeshore community, Heavenlyville area, good pay. Send CV, Box 444, *Best Journal in America.*

"Good pay." What does that mean? Would I like Heavenlyville? Classified ads are rarely specific or detailed. They are designed to generate leads, not describe opportunities. Advertisers are hoping merely to draw your response, which they then "screen" at a preliminary level so they can further investigate only the most promising prospects.

Job openings appear in general medical journals, state and county medical society periodicals, and the clinical publications in each specialty. Lead time for the ad to appear is usually four to eight weeks, and advertisers often let the ad "run" according to a predetermined schedule that spans several weeks or months. It is for those reasons that openings are sometimes filled by the time you see them.

Some journals are better than others when it comes to a well organized, worthwhile classified section. Historically, *JAMA* and the *New England Journal of Medicine* contain the most extensive listing, covering all specialties. Both journals now organize their classifieds into specialty specific sections, making them easier to use.

In addition to these general-audience journals, you might want to check the publications in your specialty reputed to have the best classified sections. For example, for radiology it is *Radiology,* for family practice *American Family Physician,* for pediatrics *Pediatrics,* and for internal medicine *Annals of Internal Medicine.* The orientation and general utility of the classifieds in one or another specialty-specific journal vary. Some tend to represent more academically-oriented job openings, whereas others tend toward more community-based opportunities. Compare the classified sections of all the journals that carry ads in your specialty. The most appropriate sources for the kind of position you have in mind should be readily apparent, even with the limited details in these ads.

Evaluating and pursuing the opportunities represented is the difficult part. You will have to devote much of your time to phone calls, letter writing, credentialing, and probably traveling around for on-site interviews. You can save yourself time here by learning to "ballpark" during the opening phone conversation. Ballparking is checking the opportunity in the most general way to see if it is roughly what you are looking for.

For example, perhaps the advertised salary is $85,000 to $100,000, a range acceptable to you, but substantial vacation time is a key issue not addressed in the ad. Therefore you call to find out, at least approximately, how much time off comes with the package. You may also want to "feel out" their attitude about associates wanting to trade income for free time. That is ballparking. If the answer is two weeks, you go no further. If it is six weeks, you talk some more.

The critical issue for you may be anything: tail coverage for your malpractice insurance, a kosher delicatessen in the community, or an intensive care unit that needs personnel so your spouse can find work too. Perhaps you want reassurance that you will have an adequate referral base for your specialty. You can and should get that information during the first phone call.

Advertisers may or may not identify themselves in a classified ad. Those who do may or may not answer questions during a first-contact call. They may want you to apply formally first, so they can devote their time on the phone to qualified applicants.

Limit your ballparking questions to items that, if the answers are unsatisfactory, would virtually rule out further discussion. Settling those issues is all you should try to accomplish before investigating in more detail through follow-up calls or meetings. The idea is to ask all essential questions but not to clutter the conversation with issues that can wait. Initial phone calls are not for negotiating; they are for gathering information, based on which you decide whether to pursue the opportunity further.

Although you may screen dozens of ads while ballparking, it is better than crisscrossing the country to interview for positions you quickly realize are of little or no interest. The nature of job hunting through classified ads is to let your fingers do the walking, to do as much "legwork" as you can by phone.

Encourage everyone with whom you speak to send material about the opportunity offered and themselves. Although this information tends to be self-serving and should be reviewed critically, it may communicate a great deal about the group or institution and the opportunity they have available. Do they send classy, well organized material or hastily compiled bits and pieces? Does it convey key details, or does it gloss over important matters? Does it communicate or obfuscate? The initial promotional material for a job rarely makes or breaks its appeal, but it can provide an early, easily obtained picture of the position and your prospective employer at no cost or obligation to you.

The key to using classified ads successfully is to take the initiative and sustain it. Take the time and energy to evaluate the opportunity, present yourself effectively, and drive for closure once you decide the opportunity is suitable.

Society and Residency Program Placement Services

With rare exception, medical placement bureaus or services are "listings" not "services." Reserved for members of the sponsoring society or college, they provide lists of job seekers and job openings to members who request them. Sometimes you must even be a member to post your opening, which severely curtails the range of opportunities represented.

As with classified ads, these listings provide no counsel, no information beyond what is in the listing itself, no assurance that the opportunity is still open. These services work on a noncompetitive, nonprofit basis, with the lack of zeal you would expect when there is no incentive to place you.

These services are not to be demeaned, but they should be viewed realistically. The listings themselves are nothing more than sophisticated classified ads that appear on the society's lists rather than in a journal. Evaluating the opportunity and, later, getting hired is based entirely on your initiative and that of your prospective employers. The passive nature of most such placement services—from that of the American Medical Society (AMA) to those of the smallest county societies—is usually a reflection of their status as unimportant departments of large bureaucracies.

Comparable in utility to the society placement services are the placement services run by many residency programs. They usually take the form of a bulletin board where opportunities are posted, supplemented by informal networking. Not uncommonly, one or another key person in a given training program becomes the de facto placement counselor for that program (it could be the chief resident, the program director, or the chairman's secretary). Such persons may have knowledge of opportunities available, so do not be afraid to ask around to determine who knows what.

Networking, or pursuing leads through key people in your residency or fellowship, should prove most valuable for finding jobs in the vicinity of your program or with its alumni. Make your interests known to your program's de facto placement counselor, and always express your gratitude for leads, even those that end in disappointment. Keep your eyes and ears open—you might find a diamond in the rough.

Private Placement Services

Terrible things have been said about "headhunters," some of which may be true. If you deal with a private placement service, it goes without saying that you should determine that it is reputable and effective.

Presuming you have done that, I recommend that you use a headhunter agency instead of (or in addition to) the nonprofit services mentioned above. There are three reasons. First, motivated people, many of whom are experienced professionals, will be working in your behalf. You, on the other hand, control the game and can evaluate opportunities without obligation or cost beyond your time and effort.

Second, a good agency does the bulk of the early investigation on both sides. There is a strong correlation between the quality of a placement service and the extent to which it knows both you and the opportunities it presents to you. With some well thought out questions, you can have a good picture of the opportunity even before you talk directly with the practice members.

Third, *it is free.* Why wander into the job market by yourself when you can have someone take you by the hand, scout the scene for you, put a network of contacts at your disposal, help you avoid the pitfalls, steer you toward what suits you, and not ask for a dime?

The institution or group that hires you pays the tab. It is important for you to be aware of this fact because, as with the real estate business, the agency primarily represents the seller, the side that pays them. However, this situation is not incompatible, and ideally is consistent, with representing your interests effectively. The agency does its job best when it creates a win-win situation where both sides get what they are looking for.

There are two methods by which search firms are paid: retainer fees and contingency fees. Some firms do contingency work only, some work only on retainer, and others do some of each. I recommend firms working on retainer but certainly not to the exclusion of those working on contingency. Be sure to ask about this point because you can then better understand what to expect.

A retainer is just part of the fee for doing a job, the part that is paid in advance. The remainder of the placement fee and the expenses incurred by the agency are paid according to some prearranged schedule. Often a substantial portion of the fee, perhaps one-third, is withheld pending satisfactory completion of the assignment.

The up-front fee commits both the agency and its client to the task at hand. The client believes that the search firm will do the job well, using its networking capabilities, advertising, and other strategies and resources. With the retainer in hand plus the client's commitment to pay for reasonable, approved expenses, the search firm can investigate the opportunity thoroughly and search for candidates assiduously. In other words, the search firm ideally can concentrate on doing the job well, not just quickly.

Under a contingency arrangement, the agency gets paid when it fills the position; it does not get paid if it fails. This arrangement is similar to the way a plaintiff's lawyer is paid in personal injury litigation. In theory, the contingency setup might seem better because the client pays only for positive results. The search firm, however, is working on speculation, under pressure to either fill the job or take a financial drubbing.

The recruiter at a contingency firm describes a position to you and asks if you are interested in pursuing it further. If so, he sends you for an interview and hopes you are hired. The problem is that he can provide any number of candidates for a given opening, hoping that one finds the situation suitable and vice versa. Sometimes, all he has done is find your name and number, leaving his client to evaluate, pursue, and "close" you.

A firm working on retainer is being paid, in part, to save its clients time and effort. Their recruiters should do more screening and credentialing than recruiters working for contingency firms. Therefore you can expect, at least in theory, that the opportunities they present will fit you reasonably well.

Although I generally favor retained searches for the reasons mentioned, each arrangement has its place. On one hand is the practice in an area for which it is difficult to recruit that has specific ideas about the physician it wants to hire. Perhaps it is looking for a female obstetrician-gynecologist from a top training program with three to ten years' experience. Such a recruitment challenge would almost certainly have to be solved on a retainer basis because no search firm would take such a difficult assignment on contingency, given the time, effort, and investment needed to fill the requirements. On the other hand, a practice with an opening in high demand among physician jobseekers, e.g., an internist position in a wealthy suburb with high guaranteed income and limited demands on personal time, would probably find several firms eager to take the assignment on contingency. Such firms already have on hand, or could readily develop, a list of appropriate candidates.

Some placement firms require an exclusive commitment from you, but otherwise there is no limit, ethical or otherwise, on the number of placement firms with which you can register. For your own sake, though, it makes sense to limit the number. If you paper the world with your curriculum vitae you may find two or more firms bringing the same opportunity to your attention. Having to decide which firm should represent you for a given opportunity is awkward; moreover, if several firms find themselves offering you the same opening, it reduces their motivation to work in your behalf. The grapevine is reasonably effective within this industry, so expect that sooner or later the firms will discover your modus operandi. Think how you would feel about a patient who not only seeks the occasional second opinion but regularly makes appointments with nearly every physician in town.

There is no formula for choosing a search firm other than to ask questions and use your own intuition about them. There are large, sophisticated firms with national scope, as well as numerous small organizations with local focus. Different firms have different strengths. Ask about their areas of concentration: A geographic area such as the upper Midwest? Small groups in rural towns or large groups in major cities? Primary care specialties or hospital-based positions?

In the absence of strong recommendations from colleagues, you may have to let your impressions guide you. Does the firm seem to be organized, professional, caring? Do their people prattle or provide you with useful information? What sort of questions do they ask? Do they seem to take a genuine interest in you? Understand your point of view? Do they respond to your concerns? Recognize your needs?

Once you have registered with one or more search firms, it is in your best interest to let their staff get to know you as well as possible. The more forthcoming you are with your "consultant" the better he will understand your preferences and the more likely he is to fill them precisely.

For example, perhaps you would be uncomfortable practicing in an office attached to a hospital building because you would feel beholden to the institution. This sort of information is usually not easily forthcoming, and a recruiter may discover it only after several interviews—another reason to work with a small number of such firms. If you register with seven or eight firms, you can plan on getting beyond the initial screening with only three or four; and often these recruiters never get to know you well enough to elicit information important to the placement process. As a result, they would send you to interview with poorly fitting opportunities, wasting both your time and theirs, and they would probably soon tire of you.

Perhaps a placement consultant has found the "perfect" opportunity for you, but you never mentioned that private schools are critical to you and your spouse. It makes no sense for you to wait until the final interview to ask, "Where are the private schools?" They could be 50 miles away, a fact that would have eliminated consideration of this job at the beginning had you been more forthcoming. If you could not be happy without a kosher delicatessen, a Latter Day Saints church, a theater that specializes in foreign films, or anything not to be found in most communities, be sure to include that information in your list of requirements.

Try to be as explicit and detailed as possible about what you are looking for. Providing good information does not guarantee that you will find what you want, but not providing good information virtually guarantees that you will not find it. In addition, make sure the firm knows they need not bother you with questionable options just to impress you that they are doing something.

Of course, you may not know what you want. If so, be frank about it. A good recruiter can draw you out and help bring your preferences into focus. It may be the first time anyone has talked with you at length about such things, and you may find that it helps immeasurably. In fact, if you do not get such attention and assistance, you might think about reevaluating the recruiting organization.

Make yourself easy to deal with. Be willing to work with the search firm in a conscientious, cooperative way. Return their phone calls, respond when you say you will, and do not procrastinate when they ask you for something. If they line up an interview, go at the earliest reasonable time. If they need your decision about a specific opportunity, do not take six weeks to give it to them. Be professional, be committed, and give them a good chance to earn their fee; it helps keep them motivated and working in your behalf.

Targeting and Networking

You are an internist, you would like to practice in San Francisco, and you want to find a group that offers a 50-hour work week with limited on-call responsibility. "Fat chance," would be the response of almost any medical placement professional. "Come back when you can be more realistic." It is a tough order, especially if you did not graduate from a training program in that area. However, people do work in those practices. How did they get there? How can I get there?

These openings are usually filled by word of mouth, through the "old boy" network. Networking is, in fact, a time-honored method of securing a practice, and it works most effectively when you know just what you want.

The essence of using networking effectively is to bring yourself to the attention of the established physicians in a favorable way. You can simply introduce yourself, of course, but it is more common and effective to gain entree through someone who knows you and your target; such introductions also serve as implied recommendations. If no immediate opening results from that contact, you at least have another "old boy" chatting the network in your behalf.

If you cannot manage an introduction, it is also reasonable, if less promising, to approach your target directly: Send a curriculum vitae with a letter of introduction. State that you are aware of the practice and that it is the kind of professional situation you have in mind; therefore you are presenting your credentials for their consideration, now or in the future.

Such communication is a long shot, but your letter could be timely. If they have an opening or have been considering recruiting a new associate, there is a chance they will be interested in you, especially if your background and credentials resonate with their requirements. If they do not have an opening, you are now in their file for future reference. They might even mention you to a colleague who is trying to fill an opening. Keep in mind that, with time, all practices change. There is virtually no practice anywhere that "never" has an opening. The idea is to make yourself known to your target practice and be available when it has an opening.

In today's world word processors have made large scale letterwriting easy, and so it is neither time-consuming nor expensive to contact numerous prospective employers. Many word-processing programs have functions that allow you to merge a standard letter with a list of names and addresses. All but the least sophisticated computer allows you to personalize the letters so you do not have to make do with the tell-tale "Dear colleague." The point here is that even if you do not know people through whom you can network, you can still present yourself in a dignified, personalized way to a large number of target practices with relatively little time and effort. For the lazy or more well-to-do, there are also direct mail firms that can do the work for you and can target your mailing to specific areas. These methods can place you in direct view of many prospective associates.

Locum Tenens

Only on the scene since the early 1980s, nationwide locum tenens groups provide physicians with a unique new way to enter the job market. Temporary associations—arranged when an established practice needs additional staffing to cover vacationing partners, vacancies, or periods of peak activity—provide a convenient vehicle for prospective associates to "try before they buy." The underlying principle, of course, is that both sides can make a better decision by knowing more about each other.

Alternatively, you can arrange a temporary placement yourself, which works well if you can get reasonably priced malpractice insurance for a few weeks or months and you are willing to deal with the business and legal details. Whether you arrange a temporary association yourself or have an organization do it for you, the important thing is to work elbow-to-elbow with your future partners before you make a long-term commitment. Direct experience is the best way to test the water and experience the all-important chemistry of the relationship.

The locum tenens job-seeking strategy works particularly well for certain situations: You know what you want and use locum tenens to network and establish contacts in areas of particular interest; you know what you want but it is difficult to come by, so you use locum tenens to "warehouse" yourself and wait patiently for your preferred opportunity to materialize.

Perhaps you have no earthly idea what you want. You are in a complete muddle about what you want in a practice or a location because you have been so immersed in training or in another practice that you have had no time to think about the future. You have limited or no experience in the "real world" and have only a dim idea of what different practices or communities have to offer. In short, you might not recognize a good opportunity if it presented itself.

Recognizing your lack of job-hunting sophistication, you stay flexible and opt for a year or two of locum tenens work. You agree to work directly for a locum tenens firm that places you in various situations around the United States for several weeks to months at a time. The best organizations can arrange work in whatever type of practice or part of the country you prefer, so long as your preferences are characterized in reasonably broad terms. Even the largest and best firms cannot arrange work for you exclusively in "the Chicago suburbs" or in "central Colorado." If you contract with such an organization for a year, for example, you can probably expect to work primarily in the "upper Midwest," or "New England," or the "Rocky Mountain states."

As noted earlier, you can also arrange locum tenens work yourself, without a professional firm. Developing a schedule, obtaining malpractice insurance, collecting fees, and arranging travel, housing, licensure, and hospital privileges can be cumbersome, however. Therefore arranging locum tenens opportunities on your own tends to work best when you work for a very limited number of clients or confine yourself to small area, thereby minimizing at least the insurance and travel hassles.

Let us say that you use locum tenens to make the transition from training to private practice.

> Your first job is with a mismanaged, disorganized practice in a city you simply do not like. However, because it is your first real-life practice experience, you may not realize what a third-rate operation it actually is. You work hard, accommodating to the problems and the difficult people; you learn what you can, and at the end of the assignment you move on.
>
> Your next locum tenens is in an equally poor practice situation but a different city. You like the area, feel comfortable there, make a few friends, and feel sad about leaving at the end of your six-week assignment.
>
> Your third stop is in a nondescript, unappealing area, but it is an ideal practice. Modern, efficient, and smoothly run, it is full of happy, high-caliber professionals who make working there a joy. This place stands out in such bold relief from your first two experiences that it knocks you over. You are not sorry to leave the area but can hardly tear yourself away from the practice.

You have learned much about yourself and your likes and dislikes after only three short assignments. Each one was far less than ideal in terms of what you are looking for long term, but you have experienced three communities and found one that you liked; furthermore, you have gained an informed perspective on the type of practice you would prefer and the type you should avoid. You have learned as much from the negative experiences as from the positive one. Even this brief odyssey has made you a more informed job hunter.

After a year of locum tenens experience, you have immersed yourself in a number of places and practices. Your former muddle has probably given way to a clearer vision of where and how you want to practice, as well as what you want to avoid. Most importantly, your assessments are based on your own experience, not the evaluations and reports of others.

Even though this approach to the job market forces you to begin the "traditional" portion of your career later than your classmates, you know much more about what is available to you and with what you must contend. You are in a position to make an informed career decision based on a foundation of empirical information. Moreover, your curriculum vitae has remained clean, unmarred by false starts or failures, you have been spared the cost of making a mistake (see Chapter 2), and you have learned a great deal about how practices operate.

Whether you use locum tenens to make the transition from training to private practice or from one practice to another, the net effect of this strategy is that it puts you in a position to pick a practice knowledgeably. There is also another advantage: You have left footprints and impressions, presumably favorable, in your areas of interest. Several groups have become familiar with you and your work. One of them may even have an opening. When they do, chances are they will contact you before searching elsewhere. You are now part of their old boy network.

It is the policy of most locum tenens firms to allow physicians to take permanent positions with their clients—for a placement fee, of course. You can expect the fee, almost invariably paid by the client, to be comparable to or less than the placement fees charged by the headhunters. Thus you can use locum tenens as a your principal job-hunting vehicle or, more likely, as an adjunct to your other efforts.

As alluded to earlier, locum tenens is also a good way for physicians to "warehouse" themselves while waiting for the right situation to come along. It is an acceptable way to maintain your skills and your income, and it relieves the pressure of having to make a hasty decision "just to have something."

The "warehousing" feature of locum tenens may be particularly relevant to physicians completing training or an employment contract on the usual July 1 along with everyone else. Competition is keen at that time of year, especially in desirable, physician-dense areas fed by numerous training programs. You are selling in a buyer's market. If you do not find a suitable opening, you can still keep yourself available. Perhaps by February the pendulum will be closer to the seller's end of the market; a senior partner may retire or become ill unexpectedly; another partner may get divorced and leave the area; the practice might even suddenly need more physicians because it wants to accept patients from a newly formed preferred provider organization (PPO).

No person or practice is invulnerable to change, and sometimes there is significant change from one month to the next. Suddenly, your ideal practice needs an associate. If they know about you and you are available, you may get the nod. By doing locum tenens and not locking into anything long term, you have placed yourself in a position to get the job despite the glut of physicians in your area of greatest interest.

Finally, the locum tenens experience itself affords you the opportunity for a life style far different from that associated with training or with a "single site" practice. Specifically, you may take free time between assignments to catch up on things you have postponed for years in order to fulfill professional commitments and career advancements.

A locum tenens period in your life can be a good time for you to "come up for air." It can be viewed as a career break or semisabbatical—good preventive medicine against burnout or frustration. It makes good sense to do locum tenens during any period of transition. The free time and flexible scheduling that are part and parcel of this type of work allow you to look around, take stock, and, ideally, find out more about who you are and what you want out of life before locking into your next major, long-term commitment.

7

How to Evaluate Specific Opportunities

Medical school taught us about clinical syndromes so we could recognize them when afflicted patients walk in the door. The same working knowledge of medical practices can help you ask intelligent questions and evaluate and compare the practice opportunities you are considering.

Five variables, based on readily available facts intrinsic to the practice, are useful for characterizing medical practices: size (number of physicians), specialty mix, legal structure, method of payment, and method of sharing expenses and dividing income. These variables address the "structural" realities of the practice. For the most meaningful and complete characterization of a situation, however, you must look at these factors in conjunction with those that are external to the practice (e.g., the history and politics of the community and the regulatory climate of the venue) as well as the more subtle, difficult to discern "functional" realities of the practice (e.g., the personality of key members and the chemistry among them, and the professional autonomy afforded the physicians). This chapter examines these important factors with comments, caveats, and points to which you should pay special attention when scrutinizing a practice.

Practice Size (Number of Physicians)

A practice can range from one end of the spectrum, where there is a single physician, to the other, where there are well over a hundred partners and associates. The demands placed on individual practice members and the benefits offered to them vary as a function of practice size.

At one extreme, a solo practice places high demands on your time but affords you complete autonomy. If a structured work schedule with limited, well defined hours is a priority in your life, you had better learn to live with less autonomy, perhaps a great deal less, and to function in some type of group setting.

Generally speaking, there is a rough correlation between the size of an organization/group on the one hand and the rules, structure, centralization of authority, availability of ancillary services, collegial support, cross-referrals, and consultation on the other. As detailed in chapter 4, there are both advantages and disadvantages that accrue with size; so make sure that a practice has at least a fair share of advantages for its particular size. For example, if you accept the limitations of practicing in a larger group, you should also look for the support that comes with first-rate ancillary services and colleagues with skills that complement your own.

Specialty Mix

SINGLE-SPECIALTY PRACTICE

Regardless of the size of the practice, single-specialty groups are generally less complex and problematic than multispecialty groups. There are fewer disagreements over dividing income in a single-specialty group, for example, because it is less complicated to compare one physician's production, contribution, and "market value" with those of another. It is usually easier as well to achieve a meeting of the minds among members of a single-specialty group on potentially contentious issues (e.g., allocation of overhead, income and on-call responsibilities, style of practice) than it is with widely divergent specialists.

As the number of colleagues in the same specialty increases, there is a greater opportunity for complementary subspecialty training and sharing of interests, improving the utility of consultations. Physicians in the same specialty have like needs and expenses as well. Conversely, in a multispecialty practice a radiation oncologist might want a linear accelerator, whereas a family practitioner needs only examination tables, good lighting, and the basic equipment he would carry in his bag or pocket. It is easy to see why single-specialty groups have much less trouble reaching agreement on appropriate investments in equipment.

Single-specialty groups are not immune from hassling over issues such as how best to divide income, however. In some single-specialty groups, for example, colleagues often refer, formally or informally, the most complex and challenging cases to the brightest and most experienced physicians in the group. These physicians are in many ways the strength of the group, but they may not generate as much revenue as the others because they see fewer, albeit more complex, time-consuming cases, and there is a limit to the amount of money they can bill for the time they spend.

A single-specialty situation also makes it easier to structure cross-coverage and on-call responsibilities. If a nine-person multispecialty group has one pediatrician, he may be reluctant to share call with the group's three family practitioners. In a seven-person pediatrics group, though, he would almost certainly be comfortable sharing call with his six colleagues.

The compelling reasons outlined above explain the domination of single-specialty groups in the United States. Over the entire landscape of medical group practices, they account for 70%.

MULTISPECIALTY PRACTICE

Multispecialty groups offer their own advantages and drawbacks, their own trade-offs. The primary-care staff provide the specialists with a built-in referral base and in return receive direct and immediate feedback from specialist colleagues they know and trust. Furthermore, they have less worry about referring a patient outside the practice and not getting him back.

On the average, multispecialty groups are larger than their single-specialty counterparts and are therefore in a position to benefit more from the economies of scale and suffer more from the disadvantages of size. They also are better able to afford managerial staff as well as ancillary services and personnel.

Compared with single-specialty groups, the drawbacks of multi-specialty group practice include a higher potential for disputes over income distribution (the most contentious issue for any group) and on-call responsibilities. Also, it is not unusual in large single- or multispecialty groups for the colleague who manages (or oversees) the business end of the practice to slip out of the clinical production loop. If he is paid only according to the clinical revenue he produces, he probably feels underappreciated and underpaid; conversely, if he is paid an additional salary for his administrative work, other partners might object.

The dispute over income and on-call responsibilities between primary care physicians and the procedure-oriented colleagues to whom they refer is age-old, as is the dispute over how much primary care one or another specialist can or should be doing. These questions have been with us for decades and will likely remain for decades hence. Multispecialty groups are the traditional battlegrounds for these disputes.

The key point here and throughout this chapter is that there is rarely a good way or a bad way to structure and operate a medical practice. On each and every issue opinions and preferences vary, depending on your or someone else's perspective and values. In terms of assessing specific professional opportunities, your main goals are to understand what you are looking at and recognize its strengths and its limitations. It is only with this background that you can decide *beforehand* how comfortable you will be with the group and its approach. In other words, *do not let yourself be blindsided.*

Legal Structure

There are three basic legal structures that apply to a medical practice: sole proprietorship, partnership, and corporation.

A practice that is *sole proprietorship* is owned by one person; the term does not connote a solo practice. A sole proprietorship can be a 50-person group, provided ownership is in the hands of one person. That individual has complete authority unless he delegates it, and he is entirely responsible for the group's obligations. Physicians who work for the practice as employees or independent contractors have professional responsibility for themselves and those they directly supervise, but they have no investment in or financial liability for the practice.

Most physicians think of a *partnership* as two physicians working together. As a legal term, however, partnership has nothing to do with size; a partnership can have any number of partners and any number of employees. Many of the giant Wall Street investment firms, for example, were until recently structured as partnerships (many have now gone public), and many large law and accounting firms still encompass hundreds of partners.

From a legal perspective the most important point for you to know is that a partnership in some ways is not a legal entity distinct and separate from the partners themselves: It makes no profit, pays no taxes, and incurs no losses. Only the partners, as individuals, do. If there is a profit or loss, it is passed on to them personally; all financial and other liabilities incurred by any one partner, including in some states medical malpractice liabilities, become the personal responsibility of all partners.

A *corporation* is owned by shareholders. In return for their investment in the corporation, as represented by the number of shares purchased, the owners may receive dividends as determined by the board of directors, which is entrusted to represent the shareholders' best interests. The treatment of corporations is different from that of partnerships with respect to both legal and tax matters. The rationale is grounded in the legal concept that a corporation, unlike a partnership, *is* a distinct legal entity for most purposes, separate from its owners. It generates revenue, makes a profit or loss, and pays taxes.

Partnership income passes directly through the business to the partners who own it. They pay tax on it one time, as personal income at the applicable rate. The partners thus avoid paying taxes at two levels, as they might have to as owners of a corporation: The corporation itself is taxed on its profits, and then the after-tax profits, if any, are passed on to shareholders as dividends, which are then taxed as personal income. Alternatively, after-tax earnings may remain in the corporation as "retained earnings," which can be used to buy real estate, equipment, automobiles, or whatever. Such acquisitions go on the books as corporate assets and contribute to the "net worth" of the corporate entity and therefore to the value of the stock held by its shareholders.

Whether it makes more sense for a corporation to distribute or retain earnings is a complex question. Probably the biggest single factor is the top marginal tax rate on corporate versus personal income. When the corporate tax rate is favorable compared with the rate on personal income, shareholders favor retaining income in the corporation and buying as much as they can with corporate profits, all other things being equal. When the reverse is true, shareholders who work for the corporation seek to minimize corporate earnings by maximizing their salary, bonuses, and other benefits, thereby avoiding "double" taxation.

In a partnership, managerial responsibility falls on the partners, who designate one partner, often called the managing general partner, to assume those responsibilities. The managing partner may then delegate managerial authority to professional managers if he deems it appropriate.

In a corporation, managerial responsibility ultimately lies with the board of directors. A board usually consists of owners of the corporation or their representatives. It generally includes members of the corporate management team as well as people outside the corporation who are neither owners nor members of management. Unlike partners, shareholders have no managerial responsibility or liability simply by virtue of their status as owners. They may assume such responsibility and liability by joining the board, taking an executive position, or both.

In the medical world one type of corporation is of particular importance—the *professional corporation*. All states have laws regulating the "corporate practice" of medicine. The laws say, in effect, that no one but a physician can practice medicine. If a practice is structured as a corporation and therefore viewed under the law as a separate entity providing professional services, it technically must be a professional corporation, which means that it is owned solely by physicians licensed to practice in the state where the corporation is chartered. These entities—professional corporations (PCs) or professional associations (PAs) as they are known in some states—operate under the authority of the state's medical board and are exempt from the canons against the corporate practice of medicine. Thus physicians form such entities to benefit from structuring their practice as a corporation without running afoul of state law.

Another entity worth considering is the *S corporation*, a cross between a partnership and a regular, or C, corporation. Like a regular corporation, the S corporation is a distinct legal entity owned by its shareholders. It is taxed like a partnership, however. The owners (shareholders) avoid the legal and financial liabilities associated with partnerships and avoid paying taxes on two levels (corporate and personal) because, like a partnership, profits and losses of an S corporation are passed directly to the owners. In short, an S corporation has the legal status of a corporation but is taxed as a partnership.

Comment. How you apply the above information depends entirely on your perspective and your goals. If, for example, avoiding liabilities is your primary interest, you may opt for employee status. If, on the other hand, your goal is to maximize income and assets, you might seek ownership and equity, look to employ others, and accept the attendant liabilities.

Method of Payment

It is important to understand how the practice you are interested in is reimbursed by patients or third-party payers. There are three fundamental methods: fee for service, capitation payment, and payment based on cost reimbursement, often from some type of "general fund," as is the case for government-sponsored care (e.g., county or Veterans Administration hospitals and most academic institutions).

The fee-for-service method is time-honored and preferred by most members of the profession. The physician charges for services rendered, and the patient or his insurer pays the bill. In many instances the insurer—Medicare and Medicaid noteworthy among them—pays only a portion, sometimes distressingly small, of the physician's "usual and customary" fee.

The rules regarding how third-party payers handle physician billings is the subject of many books. Suffice it to say here that in fee-for-service practice the physician bills for his services at the time he provides them and collects whatever he can from whoever is responsible for paying. In some fee-for-service practices, patients are required to pay at the time of service and secure reimbursement themselves from their insurance company. The practice may assist administratively, completing forms and so on. In other practices, billing is done directly to the third-party payer.

Regardless of the billing mechanics, a practice may or may not require a patient to make up the difference between what it charges and the portion of those charges reimbursed by the insurance company. As applied to Medicare patients, this point is the infamous "assignment" issue. There are often strong feelings about accepting or not accepting assignment. In some states physicians are now subject to a ceiling on what they can charge Medicare patients—the maximum allowable charge.

By contrast, practices compensated entirely or partly based on a prepaid, *capitation arrangement* are paid a fixed amount for each patient participating in the plan. Examples range for the Kaiser Permanente closed panel, staff model HMO, which is 100% prepaid, to the growing number of independent practice organizations and preferred provider organizations, wherein each participating practice may have a small percentage of its total service capacity paid for and therefore committed in advance. If the total cost of providing care to all patients in a prepaid plan is less than the fixed amount paid for their care, the practice or the plan sponsor (e.g., Blue Cross Blue Shield, Prudential, Aetna) makes a profit. On the other hand, if costs exceed payments, the practice or sponsor loses money.

On the methods of payment issue, the key considerations relevant to choosing a practice relate to the type of financial pressure a physician is likely to experience under one or another method. In the prepaid situation, physicians operate within the realities of budgetary constraints. As such, you can expect some degree of pressure to husband resources and limit expenditures because there is no way to bring in additional revenues beyond what is established in advance by the prepaid arrangement.

In a fee-for-service practice, a person or his medical insurer pays the fees charged for services rendered, or whatever portion of those fees they choose or can afford to pay. Therefore the more services provided, the more income for the practice. There are no financial disincentives to providing services. Clinical decision-making is virtually free of financial constraints unless you choose to be sensitive to them, perhaps for the patient of limited means who pays out of his own pocket.

You may be subject to pressures in the other direction, though, because your income bears a direct relation to the amount of services you provide: return visits scheduled, tests ordered, procedures performed. You have a vested interest in doing more and ordering more, and so could be tempted to go beyond what is absolutely necessary for proper care.

Practices paid on a capitation basis can take two fundamental forms: one is where the physicians work under one roof; the other is where a central entity (Blue Cross, for example) arranges with physicians in fee-for-service practice to accept a certain percentage of their patients on a prepaid basis. The latter are called independent practice associations or preferred provider organizations.

Physicians who have some or all of their income tied to capitation payments may or may not have monetary incentives that are tied to the overall financial success of the insurance arrangement. In other words, if the sponsoring organization makes a profit from providing clinical services, it might give some sort of bonus to its participating physicians.

The third major method of payment encompasses government-sponsored care, including city, state, and federal institutions and many academic centers. With this arrangement, the practice is paid on a *cost-reimbursement basis*. The motivation here is to maximize services provided and therefore costs, which in turn maximizes income to the practice or institution, assuming no budgetary constraints, which is rarely the case. Unlike fee-for-service practice, where the financial motivation is also to maximize services and therefore income to the practice, physicians in these settings are usually paid a fixed salary and therefore practice free from financial incentive in either direction. Even here, however, one could argue that financial motivation comes to play, in that physicians who earn the same no matter what they do may have less enthusiasm for going the extra mile, whether it is adding to their daily workload or getting out of bed to admit a patient in the middle of the night.

As you can see, the economic incentives affecting practices and their physicians are determined by how they are paid for the services provided. How economic incentives affect clinical activities and decisions depends on the values and character of the organization as well as the extent to which economic pressures on the organization are augmented or attenuated by the economic incentives on the individual physician—whether physicians are compensated according to a fixed salary, productivity, or their ability to provide necessary and appropriate care "within budget."

Shared Expenses and Compensation of Members

Historically, how groups share expenses and mete out compensation comprise the most contentious problems for any group. No matter how complex or straightforward a group's method of paying its physicians, someone is unhappy, believing he is putting in more, or receiving less, than an equitable share.

Expenses are borne equally among members in most group practices, but there are many methods of dividing income. One is to divide it equally; another is to divide it based on some measure of productivity, e.g., revenue generated (you get x percent of your billings or collections) or patients seen, which may or may not be combined with other measures of achievement such as speeches made, presentations given, papers published, credentials, tenure and status in the group, or grant revenue brought in. In the extreme, expenses and revenue are both figured into the compensation formula: The group treats its physicians as a profit or cost center—similar to departments or product lines of a business—with separate cost accounting for each member or specialty group.

"Share everything," the simplest way of apportioning group earnings, has been the most popular method over the years, although it has now lost ground to formulas based on productivity. In 1973 nearly 60% of groups shared expenses and income equally, but by 1989 only 37% did it that way. Over that span of time, the proportion of groups that based physician income on individual productivity jumped from 11% to 27%.

The trend favoring productivity-based compensation is understandable when viewed against the trend to larger groups. A productivity-based compensation system makes it difficult for less motivated physicians to subsidize their income by riding on the dedicated work of others.

More recently, however, methods of payment based on capitation or diagnosis-related groups (DRGs) have set economic forces into motion in the opposite direction, as less professional activity and fewer services mean more profit for groups participating in prepaid plans. Such practices prefer to engage physicians as salaried employees, thereby eliminating their financial incentive to order more tests, do more procedures, or provide more services in general. In addition to federally employed physicians, who have always worked for a fixed income, 20 to 25% of all physicians are now salaried. The percent is almost doubled for physicians under age 40, reaching nearly 60% among female physicians in that age group.

In theory, at least, salaried physicians are immune from pressures to over- or underutilize ancillary services and are thus free to practice according to their best medical judgment. However, will their zeal as patient advocates remain undiminished when the interests of their patients clash with the economic concerns of an employer who encourages them to husband resources or withhold care? The question then becomes: How does a prepaid group balance the professional concerns and economic incentives of its physicians with its own economic interests and commitment to patients? Can it be done? Some 45% of groups now receive some of their income from prepaid arrangements, so it is no idle question.

Other Variables, Issues, and Considerations

A framework for characterizing a practice by size, specialty mix, legal structure, method of payment, and method of sharing expenses and dividing income has now been established. The next set of considerations concerns other key variables germane to assessing a practice. Examining these factors can provide the information you need to characterize more completely the opportunities you are considering.

YOUR COLLEAGUES

Broadly speaking, your dealings with colleagues is a matter of "chemistry." Because chemistry cannot be evaluated until you work with a group, you need to look for a reasonable way to assess this all-important variable in advance. In my mind, chemistry in relationships reflects compatibility of goals, values, and attitudes, both personal and professional. These items can be assessed, at least to some extent, by asking the right questions of the right people.

When you speak to your prospective associates over the phone or in person, use the time to good advantage. "Small talk" breaks the ice and warms people up, but it does not get you the information and insight needed to assess your future colleague's attitudes and philosophy on a range of important issues. For convenience, you might group these issues into life style and practice style considerations. Issues of life style and practice style never go away; in fact, they either provide the foundation for solid, long-term relationships, or they sow the seeds for undoing what may at first appear to be the most solid relationship.

To ask the right questions, you must have an agenda. Know the questions you want to ask, the topics you want to cover. It matters little whether you are direct ("Let's talk about some basic philosophical issues I believe are important to all of us") or you subtly guide the conversation toward the issues you want to cover. The important thing is to broach the subjects so you both can examine them in the cold, clear light of day.

For example, it is important to assess how immersed your colleagues are in professional and nonprofessional endeavors. In other words: How committed are they? How committed are you? Would these colleagues, for example, consider you irresponsible for expecting three weeks of vacation? Would they believe you to be "abandoning" your patients if you leave for ten consecutive days to ski in Europe or sail the Caribbean? Conversely, are they looking for fun-loving associates to distribute the workload as broadly as possible, so everyone can have two or three months off per year?

Another serious issue is the extent to which professional values take precedence over business imperatives in the group. Where is the balance for this group between making money and taking good care of people? You can glean some of this information simply by observing where a colleague takes the conversation, to what extent he talks money or medicine. You may have to complement casual observations with questions that go to the heart of the matter. If you do not address important issues, they may come back to haunt you.

When gathering information from prospective employers or associates, avoid questions likely to generate "yes" or "no" answers. Ask more revealing, informative, open-ended questions and avoid giving information that might program the response.

YOUR PATIENTS

Characteristically, a practice deals with only part of the spectrum of clinical problems encompassed by each specialty it represents. The kinds of people and the problems you are likely to see in the practice depend largely on the demographics and socioeconomic status of the patient population, the clinical interests and capabilities of its physicians, and the referral opportunities in the practice environment.

A family physician who practices in a sleepy seaside retirement community sees different kinds of patients and clinical problems than the family physician practicing in a Western mining town. One deals primarily with older patients and geriatric problems, whereas the other sees young, healthy adults and deals with obstetrics, pediatrics, and the injuries that come from working and playing hard. Both physicians trained as family practitioners, but they have undertaken totally different practices. Similarly, the orthopedic surgeon practicing in Scottsdale, Arizona or Boca Raton, Florida sees different types of people and injuries than one practicing in Aspen, Colorado or Jackson, Wyoming. Just as striking is the difference in the practice of a plastic surgeon in a private Beverly Hills hospital and the one who chooses to work in a public hospital in the depressed inner city of a major metropolitan area.

Most examples of how physicians within a given specialty can treat very different patients and clinical problems are more subtle than those cited here; but whether subtle or obvious, the issue is important. You will spend a lot of time with your patients and their problems, so make sure you will enjoy taking care of them. As with all other key issues, there is no reason to be less than candid. You fool only yourself under those conditions, and it will surely catch up with you.

MANAGERIAL STRUCTURE OF THE PRACTICE

Who manages the practice? Who decides office policy, for example? What are his attitudes toward medicine, physicians, the ancillary staff? What is his management style? How does he treat others, and how do others view him? Is he a double-talker or a doer and problem-solver? Who decides when to raise fees, buy new equipment, remodel the building, add an associate or fire one?

Your prospective group may or may not have people with business and managerial talent. If the group claims to have such talent, you still need to know the qualifications, experience, and managerial philosophy of the people who are running the show. It is not unheard of, for example, to find that a group's business manager is a former nurse or laboratory technician who got the management job because of a personal relationship and is running what amounts to a multimillion-dollar business with no training or background for the job. Thus instead of having a manager who helps and supports the practice, the group is saddled with a manager who unwittingly undermines the business.

Inquire about the relationship between the physicians and the business staff. To what extent do administrative people make decisions affecting quality of care? Are nonmedical matters delegated to nonphysicians? To what extent would you have input into practice management as a new junior associate and later as a more senior one? You may be interested in issues as diverse as the group's pricing strategy, its hospital affiliations, its ancillary services, its stained carpets and barren walls. Regardless of the magnitude of the issue, make sure that your voice will be heard if it is important to you.

To summarize the subject of managerial structure, there are two fundamental issues: (1) To what extent does managerial power lie with medical people (or their representatives) or with nonphysicians? (2) Are the managers of the practice competent? The hallmark of managerial competence is the ability to get things done, to produce results, whatever the goals or agenda. Organizations lacking such competence not only make caring for patients more difficult, they can make your life a lot less pleasant than it could and ought to be.

STYLE OF PRACTICE

A physician's style of practice is determined largely by habits and reflexes developed during medical school and postgraduate training. In a solo practice you can express your own style, and to a large extent, others must adapt to your way of doing things. In a group you will have to accommodate and adapt to the practice style of your associates and to the way they interact among themselves.

* Do colleagues care little about how their associates practice, or is peer review formal and rigorous? To what extent do you have to fear someone telling you how to practice, perhaps by virtue of clinical protocols and rigid standards for productivity and resource utilization?
* What are the consulting arrangements within the group? Do colleagues offer "curbside" consults and casual advice, or do they interact only within the structure of a formally requested consult and a written reply because that is the only way they are paid for it? Do they make you feel good about asking for help or like an idiot for not knowing the answer yourself?
* Are the medical records well organized and informative, or are they sloppy and incomplete?
* Do colleagues in the same specialty round together or otherwise meet to discuss difficult problems and interesting cases? What is the nature and extent of the group's formal conferences and committee meetings? Sometimes just determining if a group has a well stocked library and a conference room reveals their orientation to collegial interaction and continuing education.
* What are the ethical priorities of the group? How do they compare with the ethical priorities on which the profession of medicine is based?

ON-CALL ARRANGEMENT

The on-call arrangement is a major factor that can affect your life style and mental health. The "intensity" of a practice's call duty is as important as the frequency of it. The advantages of sharing call with a large number of colleagues may be offset by having a more difficult time of it when it is your turn.

A three-physician group may put you on call every three nights. However, it may also have a physician assistant who takes after-hours phone calls and refers emergencies to the emergency room at the hospital, so when you are on duty it is not burdensome. You may have only the occasional call from the emergency room physician who is admitting one of your patients.

Compare that situation to a seven-physician group that puts you on call just once every week but requires you to sleep in the hospital, man the phones yourself, and see every visitor to the emergency room, regardless how sick. Which arrangement is the more desirable?

ATMOSPHERE AND PHYSICAL ENVIRONMENT

Places have a "feel" to them, and it is important that you feel good about a place where you spend countless hours. The atmosphere of a practice affects you and your patients, perhaps subliminally but certainly powerfully.

Is the environment well appointed, or is it poorly furnished? Does the staff appear crisp and well dressed, or are they too casual for your taste? Do pictures, plants, and lighting fixtures make the environment warm and inviting, or are there bare walls and dark corners that make it cold and unappealing? Is it too obviously "designer decorated," making it stand-offish and overbearing instead of friendly and professional?

The point is that you must be comfortable in and with your environment, so it should express, at least to some extent, your taste and standards. Even if the practice cannot afford to create the ideal environment, it can create a pleasant, tasteful atmosphere.

Discuss your impressions of the environment with your associates. Determine if your taste is similar to theirs. If you are not comfortable with what you see around you, find out their degree of flexibility in terms of your making changes. What investments and alterations do your associates have planned for the future? Perhaps they would be enthusiastic about your taking responsibility for that aspect of the practice.

Whatever your taste and standards, they should be in reasonable harmony with those of your colleagues. Widely disparate opinions and inclinations on these matters could become sources of conflict. Do not dismiss them as trivial.

CONTEXT OR SETTING OF THE PRACTICE

Organizations, like organisms, interact with their environment—for better or for worse, often both. A medical practice is no exception. Every practice is influenced by numerous external forces and factors, as noted earlier. Therefore in the process of evaluating opportunities, do not neglect the broader context, or "setting," of the practice. Take a panoramic view of it.

Begin with the general regional area and its patterns of health care delivery. How broad an area you choose to consider depends in part on the population density as well as the nature of the health care resources and their distribution in the area. Then look at the community itself, focusing a good deal of attention on the hospital, which may be the single most important factor to consider outside the practice itself.

The number and kind of patients you attract to your practice may be strongly influenced by the reputation of the surrounding medical community and the hospital. If the hospital is feared by potential patients as a place likely to produce harm rather than as a source of help, you can be assured that people will inconvenience themselves to find care miles away. You may wind up wondering where the patients are.

Perhaps you, a cardiologist, find a suburban town with no one else in your specialty. It seems that you should have a clear shot at handling all the cardiology referrals. Unbeknownst to you, however, the other physicians in town are close friends of one or the other of three cardiologists in a larger town 20 miles down the road. Patients do not mind the traveling because it gives them an excuse to visit the town's shopping mall, eat in better restaurants, and go to the theater. They may even believe that it enhances their status to be seen by physicians in the regional referral center.

Clearly it is not enough just to examine the practice and the community on the surface. You must learn about the established, regional patterns of patient referral and resource utilization. You must be cognizant of regional realities because you cannot readily change them (if they can be changed at all). They will surely affect your practice, if not your survival.

Be skeptical of glib characterizations of the "medical service area" and the potential patient population on which you can expect to build your practice. Group practice managers and especially hospital administrators eager to attract physicians who can fill their hospital beds wax eloquent about their ability to attract patients from far and wide. "Our medical community will soon be a regional referral center—just as soon as we can get the right number of doctors and right mix of services." Needless to say, they are sometimes guilty of overly optimistic projections.

Obviously, there is more to the public's purchase of medical care than "availability" of services: People's attitudes and habits, regional patterns of commerce in general, and utilization of health services in particular are factors you must understand and learn to live with. Regional patterns of purchasing health care and other services are well grounded in complex factors. Become aware of those patterns and factors before making a commitment; if you do locate there, you will have to adapt yourself and your practice to them.

THE HOSPITAL

Depending on your specialty and style of practice, there are many queries you must make about the hospital. As with "regional realities," you should view the hospital as a "given," not a place you can walk in and change if you do not like it, at least not at the outset. Find out about its rules, reputation, peculiarities, and powerful people—its institutional personality.

Who owns it? Is it for profit or nonprofit? Independent or part of a chain? Justifiably or not, many physicians fear that for-profit hospitals bring pressure on them to admit patients unnecessarily and even to vary treatment based on a patient's ability to pay. If, for example, a patient is on Medicare and therefore subject to the DRGs, you may be encouraged, however subtly, to discharge him "quicker and sicker." If he has private insurance, pressure may be brought to bear in the opposite direct.

Keep in mind that what holds for the for-profit sector may be just as applicable to voluntary institutions. "Not for profit" does not mean no financial motivation. Nonprofit hospitals may strive to be successful financially, if only to minimize the subsidy of whatever group has a vested interest: a religious order, local politicians, Uncle Sam. Remember, nonprofit institutions, from the local hospital to a church, may not pay taxes, but that does not mean they do not make money, accumulate assets, and behave in many respects like any other business.

Get a sense of the hospital's institutional character—its culture—and its philosophy of care, whether its emphasis is on optimal care or maximum profits. Often the best or only way, short of working there, is to ask questions of several members of the health care team, not just other physicians. Is management responsive to needs in the area? Is it supportive of the medical staff?

How much influence can you have if you practice there? If it is a small hospital, for example, managed by a board of directors from the community, you can probably expect greater responsiveness than if the hospital is large and its management is chosen by and reports to some vice president at corporate headquarters hundreds or thousands of miles away.

The hospital is often one of the largest employers in a community, and the community is often cognizant of and sensitive to its financial condition. Is it financially well off, eager to buy the latest technology and make investments in creative and exciting new medical ventures, some of which you might want to be involved in? Conversely, is it struggling for survival, engaged in questionable activities, mounting unseemly marketing efforts to attract patients and health care dollars?

Part of your practice will include referring patients to or accepting referrals from other departments within the hospital. What is the reputation of those departments? Do they have the latest equipment and well trained staff, or is the equipment out of date and the staff tired and overworked? Are all significant findings phoned to the physician or the ward, with formal consultation reports on the chart no later than the next day, or are the results reported when the physician gets around to dictating the report and the transcriptionist gets around to typing it.

If, for example, your patient goes to surgery, will the anesthesia be given by a physician or a certified registered nurse anesthetist

(CRNA)? If a nurse, will he be properly supervised or not supervised at all? If you are an anesthesiologist, you must assess with particular care the role and power of the CRNAs.

Find out specifically how to obtain privileges. Does it take no time at all, granted by a handshake from the hospital administrator, or must you wait many months for privileges to be granted by a large committee that meets quarterly and follows elaborate guidelines. Could you be excluded because you attended school in Europe or Mexico, or because you are a Jew, an Arab, an Indian, a Philippino, or because you have not been board-certified? Exclusionary barriers can be incredibly subtle: Is the required limit for malpractice insurance so high as to be too costly for a young physician starting in practice and already in debt? Does the hospital require occurrence-type coverage, a form of insurance perhaps not available to *any* new practitioner because the carriers in the area have a freeze on writing it?

Is the hospital accredited by the Joint Commission on Accreditation of Hospitals? If so, it must comply with published guidelines for screening medical staff applications. If not, it should at least be guided by is own constitution and bylaws on the question of privileges. Request a copy of the bylaws and find out how they are applied.

Depending on the size of the hospital, the medical staff can have a "departmentalized" or nondepartmentalized" structure. The first, common to larger institutions, gives each department chief considerable influence over applications for privileges. In small hospitals, departments are not large enough to be autonomous, so the entire medical staff may have a say in all hospital affairs, including your request to join them.

What is the physical plant like? Where is it located relative to the practice, to population growth, to the particular patients you want to attract to your practice?

How is the emergency department run? Are emergency medicine specialists available to treat your patients after hours, or will you have to drag yourself out of bed for even the most minor issues when you are on call, for "unassigned" patients as well as your own?

Finally, be aware of the other hospitals in the area, their local standing and reputation. Is your hospital the preferred one in the area or the one that lives on overflow from the others?

Be sure to approach nurses, patients and townspeople, as well as other physicians with specific questions in order to get the full picture. As mentioned above, it is crucial to ask open-ended questions and avoid information that might program the response. You may have a marvelous offer from one hospital in town, only to find that it is the one no one wants to go to. By working there you would be competing with the better physicians in the community who associate with the more reputable institution. Some of you would enjoy that challenge. If not, however, it is not a burden that need be assumed. Do not put yourself in a difficult situation just because you were deficient in making adequate inquiries.

Know what you are getting into.

8

Understanding and Negotiating an Agreement

Negotiations are a fact of life. From the first time you haggled with your mother over finishing the spinach, you have probably negotiated something every day of your life. That does not mean that you are as proficient at it as you might be.

It is likely that, good or bad negotiator that you are, you have never negotiated anything as important as your employment agreement. It is best not to walk lamb-like into these negotiations. By understanding the art of negotiating, you stand a reasonable chance of getting what you are hoping for and, at the same time, strengthening the foundation of the relationship with your future partner/employer.

There are three kinds of negotiation. *Soft negotiation* entails avoidance of personal conflicts and making concessions readily for the sake of reaching agreement. Soft negotiators never hurt anyone's feelings but often emerge feeling themselves exploited and bitter from all the giving-in they have done. They seldom achieve the best possible deal.

Hard negotiation is basically a contest of wills, in which the side that takes the more extreme position and holds out longer usually fares better. The wrangling, often vituperative negotiations can leave the hard negotiator exhausted—and with a new personal enemy.

When negotiating the terms of your new medical position, the third method will serve you best. It is called *principled negotiation*. It is a formal method developed at the Harvard Negotiation Project during the 1970s and was described in the 1981 national bestseller *Getting to Yes* by Roger Fisher and William Ury (Penguin Books, New York, 1981).

Principled negotiation involves deciding the issues on their merits rather than by a tug-of war. It looks for mutual gains wherever possible and relies on fair, preset standards when interests are in conflict. It is hard on the merits, soft on the people. No tricks, no posturing. Done properly, principled negotiation rewards you with what you want and deserve without short-changing the other side, and it protects you from being short-changed as well. It is the intelligent, professional way to reach an agreement.

Principled Negotiating

Negotiating from an adversarial stance seldom works as well as negotiating from a constructive, nonadversarial position. If you and the other party take positions and insist on holding them, your egos eventually get tied to your positions. Neither of you can relent on anything, regardless of who is right or wrong, because face-saving has become more important than reaching agreement.

The solution is simple: Do not bargain over positions. Instead, learn the difference between positions and interests, and negotiate interests.

> You ask for a starting salary of $90,000. Your prospective employer is offering $75,000. Those are *positions*. The *interests* are the concerns that led to the positions. Perhaps your employer offered only $75,000 because he thinks he would be overextending himself to guarantee any more. Thus his interest is that he not be overextended. You, on the other hand, need a salary of $90,000 to qualify for a mortgage on the house you and your spouse have picked out; that is your interest.

Should you compromise on your positions, split the difference, and settle on $82,500? Obviously, that solution would satisfy neither of you. Your employer might be stretching himself dangerously thin, and you still would not have your house. In this and many similar cases, compromise means both sides lose, each getting less than he wants. With a physician and an employer the mutual defeat could doom the relationship, and it would eventually fail, even if it survives in the short run. How much better it would be if both could find a way to win.

The key to win-win negotiating is to understand what the other side wants—the interests underlying the positions—and then look for ways to satisfy both sets of interests, yours and those of the other party. Sometimes the solutions are obvious, but sometimes you must invent them.

You devise new options by making a creative leap beyond the immediate issues to find a new structure for the situation. In effect, you put yourselves on the same side of the negotiating table, with each side realizing that the key to success lies as much in satisfying the other side's interests as in satisfying its own. In the above example, you must find a way to obtain a mortgage without overextending your employer. What can you work out together?

A few negotiating tips may be helpful. First, it is often wise to let the other side make the initial offer. That way you run less risk of selling yourself short or, conversely, taking yourself out of the running by demanding too much. Second, assume that the opening figure is not an extreme one from which the employer expects to be moved very far. His opening position is probably a reasonable reflection of what he expects to pay.

Third, rely on objective data or criteria to support your position. Offer evidence that $90,000 is a typical salary for physicians in your specialty in that locale. In other words, establish a rational, objective basis for what you want. You might even agree simply to accept "market" compensation and then establish how to determine what that figure is. At the same time, be ready to respect valid data or criteria the other side presents. It should be agreed before negotiations begin that relevant data and objective criteria supersede positions, and, wherever applicable, control final determinations.

Fourth, recognize the element of salesmanship in the art of negotiating. Good salesmanship involves understanding the wants and needs of the other side, his "interests," and then creating a clear and compelling vision of how you and what you have to offer can satisfy those needs. The essence of salesmanship is conveying what you can contribute to prospective associates.

Finally, if getting the most you can from a given situation means taking advantage of the other side, do not do it: It is often inimical to your long-term interests. Being taken advantage of is seldom forgotten, so you can expect to be repaid in kind at the first opportunity. You usually are more satisfied in the long run by being fair and reasonable each step along the way. In the typical professional relationship both sides stand to gain a great deal, so it should not be difficult to achieve a win-win solution.

Having examined ways and means to negotiate, let us explore a possible solution to the example given earlier. You asked for $90,000 annual salary and were offered $75,000. Perhaps you could agree to the $75,000 as a guaranteed minimum, and together you and the employer could construct a profit-sharing arrangement that is initiated only after his overhead is covered. That agreement would satisfy his interest, as he now will not be overextended. Moreover, if business is good, there is a chance you could earn the $90,000 you wanted and more.

Your prospective employer's interests are now served. What about your interest? What about the mortgage? The possibility of earning $90,000 is not the same as a definite salary at that level; it may not impress the bank or qualify you for a loan. A possible solution is for your employer to guarantee the home loan for you at the bank. If he agrees, your interest is now served. He has little risk because should anything go wrong he still has a valuable real estate investment that may well have already appreciated in value.

The two of you, through principled negotiation, have painlessly arrived at a win-win deal: Your employer has an employee with high motivation to trigger the profit-sharing portion of the agreement, and you have a boss who wants you to be successful so he makes more money and is not left with an extra house, even though it may ultimately be profitable for him.

Negotiating interests, instead of positions, works because all interests can usually be satisfied by several possible solutions. Furthermore, shared and compatible interests often lie behind what seem at first to be opposing positions.

Principled negotiation is a valuable life tool as well. It is applicable to any situation, from a schedule of chores with your children, to a lease agreement for your practice, to the fate of nations. It will serve you well to learn it, practice it, and use it in situations other than arriving at a satisfactory agreement with your future associates. The Fisher-Ury book noted above is highly recommended reading.

Employment Agreement

When evaluating an employment agreement, you will probably have to address issues you have never heard of before, let alone understand. Admittedly, such arcane issues as vicarious liability, indemnification, noncompetition, claims-made versus occurrence insurance, defined-benefit versus defined-contribution pension plans, and so on may be sufficiently overwhelming that you leave them to your attorney.

A little insight, however, can go a long way toward helping you evaluate what your advisors are telling you and ensure that your interests are properly represented. It is a bit precarious to leave such important matters solely in the hands of an advisor—whether it is a lawyer, accountant, stockbroker, business manager—to do what he thinks best. You must make up your own mind. If you do not understand what is behind the advice given, the probability of getting bad advice or being taken advantage of increases substantially. Remember that the world is rife with greedy people. Just because you are paranoid does not mean that no one is following you!

On the other hand, you need not assume that your advisors lack scruples. Simply keep your eyes open. A bit of insight and some vital information can help you assess the advice you are getting. Keeping these thoughts in mind and recognizing that a small amount of knowledge can be dangerous as well, consider the following brief guide to selected elements that are found in many employment agreements. Use the information cautiously, conferring with trusted advisors as you make decisions.

INDEPENDENT CONTRACTOR VERSUS EMPLOYEE; VICARIOUS LIABILITY AND INDEMNIFICATION

It is not unusual for a young physician to take part in a job interview and lose sight of the practical issues. He and a senior partner discuss their concepts of quality of care, the state of medicine today, medical school "war stories." They like each other, feel sure they would work well together, and finally shake hands, each with a different idea of the terms on which they have agreed.

As a case in point, the difference between an independent contractor and an employee is not merely a technicality. It reflects a good deal about your status in the practice and therefore deserves careful attention. The key issue is one of professional autonomy and liability and the extent to which your authority matches your responsibility when it comes to clinical supervision and accountability—yours over others and others' over you.

Common law, which governs the issue of *vicarious liability*, refers to the legal tradition established by the courts based on the cumulative weight of its decisions over time—in contrast to statutory law, which is written and voted into law by legislators. According to common law related to vicarious liability in "master-servant" relationships, an employee is generally considered "under the control of" his employer. The employer therefore is construed as responsible for his employee's judgments, decisions, and actions. Stated bluntly, if an employee makes a mistake, his employer can be held liable.

Therefore you can understand why the organization that hires you may want to minimize its malpractice liability by putting some legal distance between itself and your clinical decisions or actions. It can do that to a certain extent by hiring you as an independent contractor, rather than as an employee. Such a situation is satisfactory so long as you have the right to make your own decisions. The practice then is not held liable for your work because they did not tell you what to do or how to do it—and vice versa. However, if the organization somehow participates in, guides, or otherwise controls your clinical decisions or actions, you would be foolish to set yourself up as a lightening rod, drawing all liability to yourself when others in the practice might share some measure of responsibility.

Any number of difficult liability situations may arise with respect to the people you supervise, consult with, or otherwise rely on. For example, a nurse may misunderstand your orders and give the wrong medicine or relay your instructions to a patient inaccurately. The practice may have hired a physician assistant to see nonscheduled patients and he fails to consult with you on a patient with atypical chest pain who arrests shortly after walking out the door. The senior physicians in your group may dictate lines of referral and consultation, and you get incorrect advice from a recommended specialist who turns out to be incompetent. A laboratory technologist may report an incorrect result on which you rely. The person responsible for equipment maintenance may fail to calibrate the new defibrillator, and the discharge is insufficient to convert a hamster let alone your patient.

The point is that authority must match responsibility. One's prerogative to control, either through direct orders or indirectly through established guidelines and procedures, must be consistent with one's degree of responsibility and accountability—the extent to which you can be held liable for others, or others for you. To have one without the other makes no sense, either for you or for others, clinically or legally.

Another form of legal "insulation" from vicarious liability often used in employment agreements is known as *indemnification*. An indemnification or "hold harmless" clause states explicitly that one party assumes full responsibility for paying losses arising from its negligence in a relationship where the parties might otherwise be construed as having shared liability.

There are also other issues tied to the employee versus independent contractor arrangement of which you need to be cognizant. From a tax point of view, an independent contractor is considered self-employed. As such, he is responsible for paying his own taxes, buying his own insurance, and arranging his own retirement plan. Whether this aspect of the independent contractor issue is advantageous or disadvantageous for you depends on your situation. Generally, it is advantageous. Unless an organization can offer you a truly superb package of benefits, it is helpful to be able to tailor what you want in the way of benefits, augmenting some and minimizing or foregoing others, deducting everything that is allowable as a business expense.

The emergence of "cafeteria" benefit plans in the business world reflects the reality that certain benefits are far more important to some people than to others. As an independent contractor, you can create you own package and avoid having to reconcile your needs with others. After all, a man nearing retirement has benefit preferences different from those of a young woman anxious to start a family. Nowhere is this more true than in the area of pension and profit-sharing plans, where, as is discussed below, the interests of young professionals can be diametrically opposed to their retirement-age colleagues.

Another benefit of being an independent contractor applies primarily to individuals whose income increases substantially from one year to the next, as is the case for physicians completing training. Independent contractors are self-employed, and, as such, taxes are not withheld from their paycheck; rather, they pay their own quarterly estimated taxes. The Internal Revenue Service (IRS) currently allows you to limit your estimated tax payments in a given year to an amount equal to your total tax liability for the previous year. Thus when there is a substantial increase in tax liability from one year to the next, you can postpone paying a significant amount of money to the government, which you are then free to spend or invest, at least until the day of reckoning on April 15 of the coming year when the full amount is due and payable.

The advantage of being an independent contractor is not all that clear-cut, unfortunately. There are certain taxes levied on self-employed individuals that you would avoid as an employee. Another disadvantage of working as an independent contractor, alluded to in passing, is that you must either deal with the mechanics of paying your taxes and putting together your benefits or hire someone to do it for you.

The choice of working as an independent contractor or an employee is likely to be decided for you by the legal counsel of the organization with which you are to be associated. If so, make sure you understand the implications, particularly with respect to malpractice liability. If you should become an independent contractor, ensure that you get adequate advice on how to take best financial advantage of your status.

A final caveat: If you insist on being an independent contractor, for whatever reason, bear in mind that this issue is not merely a matter of the professional or financial preferences of the parties involved. The IRS prefers that people work as employees, if for no other reason than it is more efficient for them to collect tax revenue from employers than from individuals. Not surprisingly, then, the IRS is attacking the validity of independent contractor arrangements in many industries. To be valid, your status as an independent contractor must meet the test of a broad set of carefully articulated criteria issued by the IRS. If your employer is making the decision, you need not worry; but if it is your choice to be an independent contractor (or eventually to hire others on that footing), be certain that the particulars of your situation conform to those criteria.

COMPENSATION

Salary/Benefits

Your compensation is best viewed as a package with many parts. Each part should be examined individually and then the package considered as a whole. It may be a good overall package, even if many parts are less than ideal.

The cornerstone of compensation, of course, is salary, which is often called the base, or guaranteed minimum income. There may also be bonuses and profit-sharing plans. There are perks and benefits, such as health, dental, and disability insurance, malpractice insurance, pension programs, paid continuing medical education (CME), vacations, moving expenses, and automobiles. Certain elements of the compensation package may be interesting and creative, such as the guaranteed mortgage suggested above (see Principled Negotiation).

Partnership

A common arrangement is for first-year associates to receive a salary plus benefits. Becoming a partner in the practice, a common goal, usually means being paid a share of the profits. The time to evaluate the terms and conditions for conferring partnership is at the beginning, which is when you also scrutinize the basis for distributing profits as well as power among partners.

The first consideration is to determine what a partnership is worth *financially*. Your prospective associates should be forthcoming on this issue. You can expect them to provide evidence to support their financial projections. If they do not, be suspicious. If a large amount of money is attached to partnership status, you might agree to a modest salary for a few years in return for a chance to become a partner and share the profits. If, however, you find that there is little end-of-year profit because senior partners are given large salaries and extensive perks, your initial salary should be more important to you than the fast track to partnership.

If part of the compensation is based on profit-sharing, pay careful attention to how profits are defined. Traditionally, profit means revenue minus expenses, so it behooves you to scrutinize just what is included among expenses. Lavish perks skewed in favor of senior associates, such as large pension plan benefits, can boost expenses and dissipate profits to the point that there is little left to distribute.

Make sure you are comfortable with the overall plan for income distribution. Many plans are pegged to productivity (e.g., patients seen or revenue generated), some divide income equally, independent of productivity considerations, and still others take into account such factors as papers published, speeches given, CME credits earned, or other factors only indirectly related to productivity.

The issue of partnership is usually tied up with the issue of *power-sharing* and *decision-making* in the practice. You may find it distasteful to have a fair share of the wealth but no influence on how things are done, even as a full partner. Address this issue specifically; do not assume that profit-sharing is synonymous with power-sharing.

A key issue associated with granting partnership is the terms and conditions governing the decision, coupled with the group's track record on bringing new partners into the group. Are the criteria clear and objective or fuzzy and subjective? Are they written down? What would it take to change them? Did the last four junior associates make it to partnership? If not, what happened?

Facts are stubborn things, as the Great Communicator, Ronald Reagan, has said. As with clinical decision-making, it is well to support initial impressions with the best data available. You are entitled to a reasonable comfort level and to the facts needed to achieve that level. Do not be afraid to ask.

MALPRACTICE INSURANCE

It is probably not enough to know that you are being afforded "adequate" medical liability insurance, even if you have complete faith in the entity hiring you. You must be aware of and understand several specific areas of the coverage so you can decide for yourself if it is sufficient.

There are two fundamental types of malpractice insurance: *occurrence insurance* and *claims-made insurance* (detailed in Chapter 2). Here we focus on issues germane to each, although you are most likely to encounter claims-made insurance, as most underwriters eschewed writing occurrence coverage during the mid-1980s and have remained with the claims-made form of the beast ever since.

First, you need to identify the insurance company and determine its financial status. Even the most attractive policy can be rendered worthless by a bankrupt carrier. The carrier must be there when you need it. All large, established insurance companies are rated by Best & Co. Best's ratings are to insurance firms as Standard & Poor's are to stocks and bonds and Dun & Bradstreet's to a company's credit worthiness. The Best rating is a reasonable reflection of the financial status of an insurance carrier. Small companies, such as many physician-owned "mutual" insurance outfits, "captives," or the growing variety of "risk retention groups," are not rated by Best. Because they are not rated and because many have not been around long enough for anyone to judge their underwriting policies, it is impossible to determine their financial soundness. You may thus be taking a substantial risk to be insured through them.

Given the difficulty of assessing the financial status of an insurance carrier, how do you steer clear of problems? It helps to place your coverage through large, reputable brokers such as Marsh & McLennan or Alexander & Alexander, both of which are national firms. Large, reputable regional firms also exist. A small-company insurance agent may know little more than you do, so make sure you understand the capabilities and experience of your broker or agent.

Sufficient coverage is another major question. How much is enough? The answer is based on your specialty and location. For example, $1 million/$1 million limits may be extremely generous for an internist in rural Kentucky but grossly inadequate for an obstetrician in South Florida. Internal medicine is not the high-risk specialty that obstetrics is, and the malpractice climate in Kentucky is not nearly as litigious as that in South Florida, nor are the awards as fantastic. Therefore before you agree to a level of coverage, determine the "reasonable and customary" limits for your specialty in general and, as best you can, for the location where you intend to practice.

Limits are stated in two figures. The first refers to the limit for any one incident or claim and the second to your cumulative limit for the policy period. If you have $1 million/$3 million limits, you can have three $1 million losses during that period, six $500,000 losses, and so on. If you have a single loss of $1.2 million, however, $200,000 over the per claim limit, you must assume responsibility for the $200,000, even though the cumulative limit for the policy period is $3 million.

If you are looking at a group practice, ask if the policy limits apply to each group member separately, or if they are aggregate limits for the group as a whole. With the latter, a loss incurred by one member of the group reduces, by that amount, the protection available to other members for the remainder of that policy period. If a group has $3 million in aggregate limits and one member suffers a $300,000 loss, the group then has only $2.7 million of protection until the policy is renewed.

It is increasingly common for policies to be structured around aggregate limits. The approach is acceptable, provided the limits are reasonable. With this type of policy, it is a good idea to put the group's limits into perspective by asking about their history of litigation and losses. Later, it would be to your advantage to keep a close eye on things as the policy period progresses so you can take action if it appears that the margin of safety is eroding.

Some policies contain restrictions that could further modify the limits of coverage available to you. Some include a per-patient limitation, for example, as distinguished from a per-occurrence limitation. If the same patient sues three doctors in your group over the same incident for $1 million each and wins, the policy pays a maximum of only $1 million—the group's per-patient limit—even though the per-occurrence limit of $1 million for each physician would otherwise have made available $3 million.

Another important point is the amount of the *deductible*—the "self-insured retention," or SIR. There are three key questions: How much is the deductible? Who pays it? Does it include defense costs? The latter question can be critical, as defense costs can be staggering.

The issue of the deductible amount is also important because it could set up an adversarial relationship between you and your insurer. Cynically speaking, it is in the carrier's best interests to settle any claim, regardless of merit, so long as the amount remains within your deductible. That is not to say they will, only that the incentive is there. You might make a considerable investment in defense costs, only to find the rug pulled out from under you when your carrier is presented with the option to settle within the deductible, eliminating its risk with no cost to itself.

It can be a rude awakening to find that your group has a $25,000 deductible and, according to the proverbial fine print of your employment agreement, you are responsible for "all losses not covered by the policy." You thought the phrase referred only to losses above the policy limits and, having gotten comfortable with the adequacy of the limits, you were comfortable with the policy. When it comes to employment agreements and insurance coverage, surprises rarely turn out to be good ones.

If you are dissatisfied with elements of the malpractice insurance provided by an organization, there are alternatives available other than negotiating a compromise between what you want and what they have. For example, you like almost everything about a certain practice situation except the malpractice limits. You would be the tenth physician covered by the policy, and the $1 million/$3 million aggregate limits seem inadequate for that number. You raise the subject in discussions, but one of the partners explains that the group has never lost more than $200,000 in any year. They see no need to raise their coverage limits and pay higher rates. You counter that there is no certainty the group's losses will remain below the policy limits next year.

What win-win solution can you create to resolve this problem? One answer is for you to accept the group's limits. They, in turn, agree to keep you informed about the losses and agree to let you opt out of your contract any time the group's cumulative losses in a given year exceeds $500,000 (or whatever level seems reasonable to you). Alternatively, you might buy your own "excess" insurance policy. With this type of insurance, coverage begins after the limits of another "primary" policy have been exceeded. Because a primary layer of insurance "cushions" such excess coverage, companies can offer considerable limits for relatively little cost. Despite all the publicity garnered by enormous malpractice settlements, they are not common. Most settlements and awards remain at moderate financial levels, so compared with primary coverage, excess-type coverage is a bargain.

PENSION AND PROFIT-SHARING

Pensions and profit-sharing plans are slippery issues because Congress changes the rules governing them with uncanny regularity. Therefore and because the law governing pension programs is an arcane subspecialty in the legal profession, it is especially important to obtain knowledgeable professional guidance from someone subspecializing in this area.

There are four key aspects to almost any pension and profit-sharing plan: eligibility, contribution, vesting, and whether or not it is "qualified" under federal law. *Eligibility* refers to the length of time you must be employed before you can participate in the plan. *Contribution* defines the amounts that can be put away on your behalf and by whom. The *vesting schedule* is the rate at which you actually "own" and become entitled to the money set aside for you. *"Qualified" plans* are those that conform to the federal guidelines that allow pretax contributions and tax-deferred earnings on plan investments. In addition to the obvious advantages of setting aside money before Uncle Sam takes his share and earning tax-deferred returns on your investment, a qualified plan also reduces your taxable income, which may lower your overall effective tax rate.

There are two basic types of pension and profit-sharing plans: *defined contribution* and *defined benefit*. In the former, there is a maximum annual contribution allowed under the law but no limit on how large the fund can become, depending on the annual contribution, the years of funding, and the return on investment. It can reach a healthy level if you start early, fund consistently, and invest wisely. It is the more attractive plan to a young person.

A defined-benefit plan is more beneficial to people nearing retirement. It is set up most often for a partner who neglected retirement planning until relatively late, perhaps in his late fifties. With only seven or eight years to accumulate an income for retirement, he is not interested in a defined-contribution plan because he does not have time to build comparatively small annual contributions into a large fund. He needs to make major contributions now if he is to create a fund large enough to provide him with a livable annual income during retirement.

A defined-benefit plan, as its name indicates, lets him define his benefit instead of his contribution. He may say, for example, that he wants $30,000 a year during retirement beginning at age 65, which is eight years from now. An actuary then computes the annual contribution required to achieve that benefit based on the years available for funding and the expected return on funds invested over that time. In most cases the contribution required (and allowed as pretax funding in "qualified" plans) is much larger than would be permitted in a defined-contribution plan.

Simple mathematics explains why defined-benefit programs work strongly to the advantage of the older members of a group. In fact, for the youngest members the annual contribution may be negligible, compared with those possible in a defined-contribution plan. Thus in a group practice with members at both ends of the age spectrum, a substantial proportion of the revenue generated by younger group members may be siphoned off to fund the high annual contributions of older partners in the group's defined-benefit plan. That is revenue you may never see again. Of course, you may be willing to fund the plan for senior associates, expecting that your pension will, in turn, be paid by those who follow.

The idea here is not to turn you into pension experts but to make you aware that it is not nearly enough to know that the position you are considering comes fully equipped with a pension and profit-sharing plan. You need to know enough about such plans in general and the one you are being offered in particular to understand if—and to what extent—it operates to your benefit.

FORM OF OWNERSHIP

Ownership has its privileges but also its liabilities, each of which varies depending on the legal structure of the organization. It is imperative that you understand how the organization is structured and the risks and rewards associated with your status as employee, stockholder, partner, or a combination of those positions. Read Chapter 7 carefully and then discuss the issues with your advisors.

MANAGERIAL CONTROL

Managerial control is a distinct issue, separate from ownership or employment status. Being a partner or shareholder does not necessarily give you a voice in managing the practice (see Chapter 7). Therefore if you want to be involved in management and want to have input in that area, you must address the subject specifically.

Look at the organizational chart (if there is one) and the bylaws to determine the locus and mechanism of decision-making authority. Find out how, where, and to what extent the physicians in the practice influence managerial issues. You may have control over hiring, firing and directing the nurse who handles your patients but none over the laboratory technologists or the fees, scheduling, or other aspects of practice operations.

It is also valuable to understand the group's history. Who started the practice? For what purpose and with what goal? The difference between a group founded by physicians and one founded by non-physicians (a sponsoring organization such as a hospital, a community, or a religious or business group) can be significant, particularly when it comes to the nature and extent of physician input into running the practice.

It is also critical to understand that informal authority may differ from formal authority. Thus it is important to determine who holds what informal authority, which may not be apparent from inspection of the organizational chart or practice bylaws. For example, the business manager may have little formal authority, but because he is the spouse of the senior partner he may rule the practice with an iron fist.

There are no hard rules for negotiating in this area. Managerial dynamics vary greatly from one practice to another, so you must feel things out for yourself. Ask as many questions as you must of several people, and keep your eyes open. In this way you should be able to determine who influences what and which managerial issues are open for discussion. Authority is one area in which reality may be obscured and the true picture unable to be deciphered from casual inspection. In that case, the only way of discovering the way power is distributed is to work in the practice.

TERMINATION

Termination is probably the single most important and least discussed issue associated with getting hired. You must know who can fire you and for what reasons. You also must know how you can extricate yourself if you so desire. Can a single partner capriciously dismiss you the day before you are eligible for partnership? Can you be dismissed by the medical director of the group for any reason or no reason, or can you be dismissed only for "cause," based on a majority vote of the partners?

What is sufficient "cause?" When used in this context, "cause" has specific meaning under state law. Nonetheless, its definition there may be different from the language laid out in your employment agreement. The more well defined the basis for termination is in your contract, the less vulnerable you are to the judgments or jealousies of those in a position to continue or terminate your employment.

You must be careful here. Hiring and firing decisions are almost invariably subjective to some degree. By being overly insistent about definitions and clarifications, you could raise suspicion that you are trying to bind your prospective associates to a relationship they may later have legitimate reasons for wanting to terminate.

Of all employment-related issues, the ones associated with your departure are probably the most important to define in advance. The emotions associated with terminating a relationship often preclude rational discussion of the issues at the time they become relevant. It is reasonable that a certain amount of subjectivity governs these decisions, but at least you can clarify the process in advance so you can decide beforehand if you are willing to abide by it.

In addition to defining *how and on what basis* you can be terminated, an employment agreement should address the following questions in the event of your termination:

• Who provides your tail insurance?
• Do you keep local hospital privileges, or are they automatically revoked upon termination?

- Do you get any outplacement services?
- Are there restrictive covenants on your freedom to set up a new practice?
- What happens to whatever equity you hold? Is there a buy/sell agreement defining the terms and conditions for the sale of your equity or assets?
- What happens to the money set aside in your pension plan?

NONCOMPETITION CLAUSES

Depending on the practice location, it may be reasonable for the employer who asks you to leave his employ also to enjoin you from setting up or associating with a competing practice within a limited geographic radius (e.g., five or ten miles) for a limited period of time (e.g., one to three years).

The rationale for such restrictions is that there was time, effort, and expense invested by the employer in bringing you into his practice and area. Your initial success was predicated to some degree on his reputation and endorsement as well as access to his patient population and professional connections. If you leave, therefore, he is entitled to some protection from your "using" those benefits to compete against him, or from having you take advantage of them without compensating him.

Noncompetition clauses can often be omitted if you agree to compensate your employer for not invoking restrictions should you depart the practice. The amount is negotiable; it should be fair consideration for the benefits you received by virtue of the association and/or some estimation of the costs the employer incurred in providing them.

Most states refuse to enforce unreasonable noncompetition clauses, and they have strict guidelines as to what is reasonable and what therefore they are willing to uphold in court. Some states do not sanction any sort of noncompetition agreement, but they are the exception. The question usually becomes "what is reasonable" regarding the two key elements of the noncompetition clause: length of time and area of restriction.

Unfortunately, there is no solution that suits everyone. Efforts to preclude you from practicing anywhere in the state for a period of ten years, for example, would be laughed out of court. At the other extreme, efforts to preclude your practicing within several square blocks of the practice in question for a period of six months would probably be enforced. Between those two extremes, though, it must be left to you and your employer's discretion. Judgments have varied widely. To make an informed agreement you must consult an attorney conversant with this issue and how the courts have dealt with it in the venue in question.

There is more to this issue than reasonable restrictions on time and location. When you talk to counsel on this subject, be sure to ask about the terms and conditions critical to the enforceability of a noncompetition clause for the particular venue. To be enforceable in North Carolina, for example, a noncompetition agreement must have been a condition of employment, and the agreement must have been signed before employment began. Such fine points can render useless an otherwise reasonable restriction, and you can be sure that lawyers will find such loopholes. Whether such details work to your advantage depends, of course, on which side of the issue you are.

Note that a noncompetition clause should not be an automatic turnoff. Most of us have been employees not employers, and understandably we see things from the employee's perspective. It is well to remember, though, that employers have rights and legitimate self-interests, and it is appropriate that you acknowledge and respect them.

Timing the Negotiations

As for most things in life, timing is important if not critical in negotiations. Some time between when you first say hello and the time you sign a contract, you must obtain a clear picture of what you are being offered. The most important thing is that at some point before signing you clarify the specifics and understand fully what you are agreeing to. With this priority in mind, also be aware that it is important to know when to ask what questions, when to push for what is near and dear to you, and when to back off and let things simmer.

As you might expect, there are no hard rules, only general guidelines that you must tailor to the situation at hand. Think about the interactions with your prospective associates as evolving in four phases: "ballparking," clarifying, negotiating, and finalizing.

Your initial discussions should be just that—discussions, not negotiations. Your goal should be to "ballpark" all key elements of the offer; in other words, get a general idea of what is being offered as well as the degree of flexibility, if any, on issues of particular concern to you. Phone calls alone should allow you to arrive at that point. It makes little sense for either side to invest in an interview if you have major differences on key issues. It would be difficult, for instance, to successfully negotiate a compensation differential of 100%, or for the group to employ your spouse as its radiologist when the senior partner's spouse is already ensconced in that position.

The next step is to discuss and clarify the specifics of the key issues on which you have agreed in general. This stage can be undertaken by telephone after the preliminary calls or in person during an on-site interview. The most important facet of this phase is to ascertain that the specifics DO get defined and clarified—ALL the specifics. It is your responsibility to bring up any reservations you may have. You can be rest assured that the other side will do the same.

This phase of your interactions blends into the next phase, negotiations. Part of clarifying an offer is evaluating the flexibility of your prospective associates on issues of concern to you when the particulars do not satisfy your needs. It is possible that the other side will have no problem with a change you deem critical. It is perhaps best if you test the waters gently, looking always for the "interests" behind the "position." The more difficult negotiations and those that involve the most important issues may be postponed. Occasionally, satisfying both sides with a win-win scenario for a major issue proves impossible, although total impasses occur uncommonly.

It is good practice to allow the person with whom you are negotiating to set the tone, pace, and structure of the conversation. Put him at ease and by all means avoid a threatening atmosphere. The goal is to establish a nonadversarial negotiating situation. At the same time, you will have to take the lead if the other party does not clarify points important to you or fails to address all the items on your agenda. It is good to be cordial but not so eager to please that you leave important issues unresolved.

The clarification/preliminary negotiation phase of your interaction ends when you have a reasonable written offer in hand. The elements of the agreement should at this point be both clear and specific, characterized at a level of detail appropriate to the issue. You are now at the point where value judgments play an increasing role.

It seldom makes sense to start seriously negotiating details before you are clear about the whole picture. Putting things into context generally places them in perspective as well.

Examine the overall employment agreement:

- How do you feel about the whole picture? If it is generally satisfactory, narrow your view to its specific elements.
- Is an item particularly onerous or disagreeable? How negotiable is it? How troublesome is it? What are the trade-offs? Can you envision a satisfactory compromise? What would it be? Consider the issue in the context of the whole. How tolerable or intolerable is it now? Are there other items you would be willing to sacrifice in return for improving that element?
- Is there an aspect of the deal you simply cannot accept? Have you fully explained your underlying "interests"—in contrast to your position—to the person with whom you are negotiating? How open-minded have you been when considering the interests of the other party? Have you tried to create scenarios that would satisfy the interests of both parties?

Any item that makes you distinctly unhappy at this stage will likely fester and come back to haunt either you or your associates later. If it is important, deal with it *now*. Discuss it; go as far as you can to resolve the matter to everyone's satisfaction, exhausting all win-win possibilities you can create. If you are still unable to resolve the issue, perhaps it would be worthwhile to discuss it with someone who has more experience and whose objective distance allows him to see more clearly the interests of both parties, put them in perspective, and suggest possibilities for mutual satisfaction.

Remember that you started out looking for the "perfect" practice but realistically hope to find the "best possible" one. Nothing is perfect. "Reasonable" is something the two sides must be; both you and your employer will probably make trade-offs and accept compromise. Simply make sure you can live with the final arrangement.

Remember, too, that although clarity and specificity are important, not everything must be excruciatingly detailed. If you believe you cannot trust your prospective partners to do what they say they will do, at least on issues that are virtually impossible to reduce to writing, you probably should reconsider your involvement with them. Lawyers have an uncanny ability to circumvent even the most tightly drawn contract, so if there is no foundation of trust in the relationship it probably should not be pursued.

Along those same lines, a final piece of advice is in order: Do not let your attorney conduct your negotiations. *You* are in charge, not your attorney. Lawyers can give you good advice, but their focus, understandably, is on the things that could go wrong. Your goal is to reach agreement, not necessarily to solve all potential problems. If your lawyer spots a problem, take a realistic view of it. In business— and getting a job is serious business—you cannot avoid taking risks. The issue is what risks you choose to take. Your lawyer's job is to tell you about those risks. Your job is to decide what risks are worth taking.

■ 9

Conclusion

I wrote this book to help you, my colleagues, make more knowledgeable decisions about where and how to practice. My goal was to provide a definite strategy and structure that would help you better understand who you are and what you want out of life; the types of professional opportunities available to you and the trade-offs inherent in each; where to look for practice opportunities and how to maximize the options that suit you; and how to evaluate specific opportunities of particular interest and then negotiate a good agreement.

The need for this text is engendered by the failure of our graduate training programs either to provide the diversified experience needed to choose a practice wisely or, at a minimum to make career counseling part of their training curricula. This book, any book, can do only so much to correct these deficiencies.

The best foundation for choosing a practice wisely is one's own direct experience; anything else is but an adjunct, or, at worst a poor substitute. Until the profession recognizes the importance of helping its members make informed career decisions and embarks on programs that give its youngest members experience in "real world" settings such as the ones they encounter when they complete training, the turnover rate and level of dissatisfaction of physicians in practice is doomed to be higher than it needs or ought to be.

If the motivation for reorienting postgraduate training to the real world were based solely on the benefits relative to choosing a practice, we might wait a long time for such a reorientation to occur. Fortunately, there are benefits related directly to the proper clinical training of young physicians as articulated by the *New England Journal of Medicine* in its recent call to "get medical education, or at least more of it, out of the hospital and into the outpatient clinic." The *Journal* makes the following points in favor of training physicians in ambulatory care:

> The clinician of tomorrow will be called on to exhibit skills and judgement that can be learned only in outpatient settings . . . There are whole topics of medicine, diseases, observations, actions, and decisions that are just not encountered in the care of hospitalized patients any longer . . . From this perspective, ambulatory care education is nothing more than a part of graduate medical education that has been newly valued. It is, to be specific, a social good from which all will benefit . . . Deans and faculty members must recognize and publicize the importance of ambulatory care and training. (D.D. Federman, *New England Journal of Medicine* 320: 1556, 1989)

Postgraduate training is limited or heavily weighted to inpatient management of complex problems and critically ill patients, thereby failing to prepare physicians to function effectively as clinicians outside the academic referral center where approximately 90% of the profession works. It also fails to prepare physicians for choosing a practice wisely. The solution to both problems is the same: Shift a greater proportion of postgraduate training to "real world" settings.

For the purpose of preparing residents and fellows to make better clinical as well as career decisions, the optimum strategy is for academic institutions to cultivate relationships with a constellation of practices that, taken together, mirror the universe of patients and professional settings available to physicians. Compared with the skewed training physicians must now bear, the experience of working in such settings would be clinically well rounded; it would also provide adequate opportunities for physicians to understand the advantages and disadvantages of different types of medical practice and to develop a clearer vision of where to position themselves in the profession.

These goals certainly appear laudable, worthy of embrace by every teaching institution. Reorienting postgraduate medical education along these lines would surely help physicians provide better care and live happier lives.

Finally, I want to thank all the physicians who, over the past ten years, have brought to my attention the problems, anxieties, and aspirations associated with their quest for the "perfect practice". Their experiences provided both the impetus and the foundation for this book.

Index